Baby
PROOF

Mocktails for the Mom-to-Be

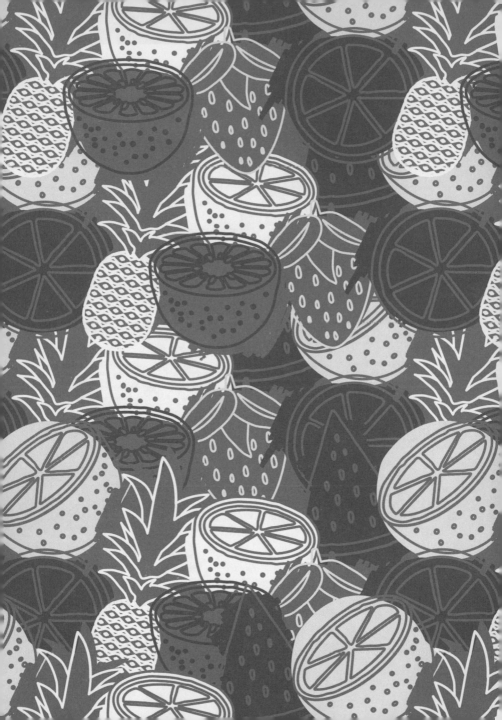

Baby
PROOF

Mocktails for the Mom-to-Be

Nicole Nared-Washington

THE COUNTRYMAN PRESS
A DIVISION OF W. W. NORTON & COMPANY
INDEPENDENT PUBLISHERS SINCE 1923

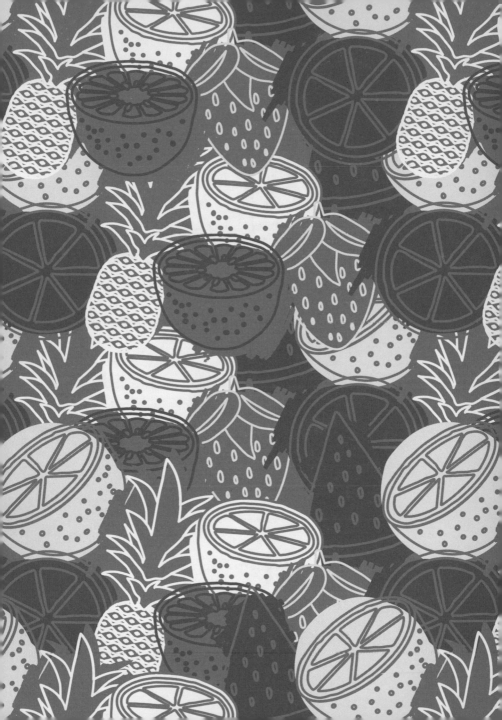

CONTENTS

From the Garden

THE FIRST TRIMESTER 25

②

Booze-Free Classics

Something Sweet

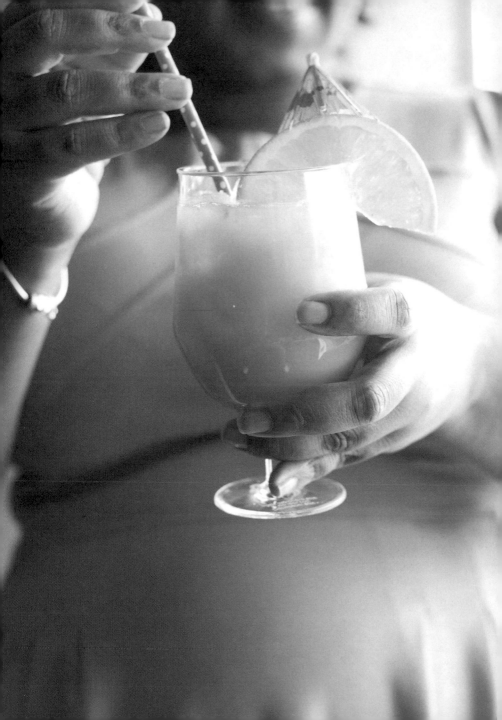

INTRODUCTION

I'M GOING TO SAY WHAT I THINK MOST PREGNANT WOMEN WANT TO SAY WHEN THEY ARE PREGNANT: "I could go for a drink right about now." Last year I gave birth to a beautiful baby boy, and all throughout my pregnancy I never wanted a drink so badly. I'm not talking about a glass of wine. I'm talking about a nice, stiff cocktail. The crazy thing is, I am not that much of a drinker. However, when I was pregnant I didn't feel that way. I know some sources say that having a glass of wine here and there during your pregnancy isn't harmful to your baby. However, my husband didn't care about those sources and, deep down, I was a bit paranoid myself. So I went nearly 10 months of my life with this craving I couldn't get rid of and nearly lost my mind!

In this book you have in your hands, you are going to experience 50 mocktail drinks that may not give you the buzz you experience in most cocktails, but you will enjoy the juice combinations that will remind you of those classics drinks such as the Cosmopolitan, Amaretto Sour, Hurricane, and Sex on the Beach, the last of which

I call Baby Momma on the Beach. You will enjoy all the flavors and the freshness of these mocktails without worrying about your growing bambino. As your body prepares itself to carry another life, it may not be that kind to you. I am sure you are enduring plenty of uncomfortable responses, such as nausea, vomiting, constipation, stretch marks, fatigue, loss of appetite, crazy cravings, headaches, and swollen feet and legs, among other things, and it would be nice to have a drink. At least that is how I felt. I am confident you will find a mocktail in this book that will ease your symptoms just by giving you something delicious to sip on. I spent a lot of time thinking about the ingredients that are used in these drinks. Here are a few rules I went with to make sure that you aren't just drinking syrup and processed sugars, but beverages that have some nutritional content and are just as yummy.

Rules of the Book

JUICE: When at all possible, make sure you are juicing your ingredients. If you are making a mocktail that needs orange, pineapple, or cranberry juice, try your best to juice the fruit fresh. I know that may be a bit cumbersome, but think of it this way: the natural juices from fruit will load your body full of antioxidants and vitamins, which are essential for a happy, healthy mommy and a happy, healthy baby. If you don't have a juicer, no biggie! Just buy your juices as natural as possible or freshly squeezed from your favorite local specialty market. You will find that not only are your beverages more refreshing, but they taste better as well.

USE FRESH HERBS: Adding herbs to mocktails can elevate the flavors to another level. Instead of a cocktail tasting like sugar, fresh herbs can add a great contrast to a beverage by making something more refreshing and delightful. Also some studies show that fresh herbs can help reduce common pregnancy symptoms, such as nausea or morning sickness, and help with labor. So, you see, I'm thinking about you!

TEA: No matter how strongly you steep your tea, it will not take on the flavor of vodka. I promise. It is going to taste like tea. However, to keep things as healthy as possible, tea is a nice alternative to alcohol. In addition, you will be adding the nutritional properties of the tea to your beverage.

STRAIN YOUR JUICE: You may notice that when you juice fresh fruits and vegetables, some foam rises to the top of the container. Because we want the freshest juice for your mocktails, there are a couple of things you can do:

- You can strain your fresh juice through a mesh strainer. This may take some time, but you can stir the juice in the strainer to help press the juice through the mesh.
- Once the foam separates, which takes only about 5 minutes after you have finally juiced your produce, use a slotted or mesh spoon and simply scoop the foam out of the container. This method works best for me and leaves me with pure juice for my mocktails.

- Place the produce in a food processor and blend. Once you have juiced your produce, you can place the juice in a food processor and blend on low speed for 5 minutes to allow the foam to emulsify into the juice. This may not take away all the foam, but it will decrease the amount of foam that is present.

HAVE FUN: The mocktails that I have created are based upon my personal sweetness level. I always encourage readers of my blog to use my recipes as a stepping stone or template to create their own deliciousness. If you know things can be a bit sweeter to you than to most people, I would start off with half of the added sugar in the recipe's ingredient list and add more as your taste buds see fit. Also, if you want more of a certain flavor, add more! If there is a flavor in a drink that you are not particularly fond of, start with less. The point is to have fun.

USE FLAVORINGS, NOT EXTRACTS: You will find that I've used rum or bourbon flavoring in some of the mocktails. The biggest difference between extracts and flavorings is that extract contains a natural ingredient, whereas flavoring is more artificial—but both can contain alcohol. Although using a teaspoon of flavoring is not likely to harm you or your baby, please conduct your own research and talk to your doctor about what is best. I should note that the flavorings I've used do not contain alcohol.

Products I Use

Here are some awesome drink mixes that do not contain alcohol that I used in creating these mocktails.

DAILY'S COCKTAILS PEACH MIX: I used this mix for Frozen Peach Bellinis and Baby Momma on the Beach.

FINEST CALL PREMIUM STRAWBERRY PUREE MIX: Used in the Strawberry Daquiri

MASTER OF MIXES PIÑA COLADA MIXER: Used in the Virgin Piña Colada

MASTER OF MIXES SWEET N' SOUR LITE MIXER: Used in Virgin Amaretto Sour

MR. & MRS. T ORIGINAL MARGARITA MIX: Used in the Frozen Margarita

POWELL & MAHONEY MOJITO SPARKLING COCKTAIL MIXER: Used in the Blackberry Mojito

PREVISTO AMARETTO- AND COCONUT-FLAVORED SYRUPS: Used in the Virgin Piña Colada and Virgin Amaretto Sour

Enjoy!

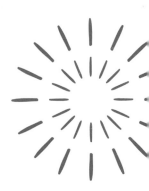

ABOUT THE INGREDIENTS

THIS BOOK CONTAINS A HEALTHY BALANCE OF INGREDIENTS THAT WILL CREATE SOME OF THE MOST DELICIOUS MOCKTAILS YOU'VE EVER HAD.

Sure, some contain artificial ingredients, and you can serve these as a treat to yourself and friends (you must live a little bit, ladies), but I wanted as much as possible to make these drinks naturally healthy for you and your baby. While coming up with these drinks, I researched many of the ingredients and how they help promote a happy and healthy baby and mommy. I was shocked by the nutritional properties and vitamins that exist in natural fruits and vegetables! Heck, if we ate enough fruit and vegetables, we wouldn't need to take huge prenatal vitamins every day! (That is not a suggestion, just a thought.) I want to encourage you to conduct your own research about some of these ingredients and discuss them with your doctor if you find it necessary. I want you to feel good about what you are drinking, and I didn't put anything in this book that I wouldn't have tried myself. But please use your

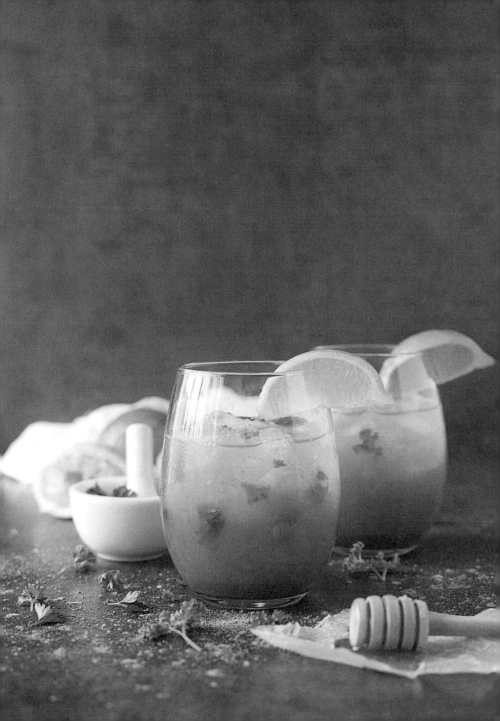

own judgment. Read on as to the nutritional benefits these fruits and vegetables have that are great for you during your pregnancy.

BEETS: This earthy-tasting root vegetable has become one of the hottest superfoods of the past decade! Beets have many wonderful properties that are beneficial to our overall health and can make for a happy and healthier mommy during pregnancy. Beets are a good source of iron and are rich in folic acid, which is extremely vital to babies before, during, and after they are born. Folic acid helps reduce birth defects and is essential for regular tissue growth and a baby's spinal cord development. Along with that, beets can help prevent anemia, regulate the metabolism, boost the immune system, and for those inevitable leg cramps that occur in the last trimester (I had those, ugh!), beets can help with joint pain and serve as an anti-inflammatory to reduce those suckers.

BERRIES: You will see quite a few mocktails with berries in this book. That is because berries are super yummy and full of antioxidants, which are important during pregnancy. The fiber from berries can also help relieve constipation and the development of hemorrhoids, which no one wants to experience. Berries are also packed full of vitamin C, potassium, and folic acid, which is an important nutrient that can help reduce the risk of birth defects.

CARROTS: Babies come into this world with the most beautiful and softest skin. It has been untouched and unscathed by the environmental elements they will experience outside of the womb. Carrots help support our babies' skin while they are inside our belly. The nutritional properties of carrots are great when it comes to supporting your unborn baby's skin and muscles. In addition, carrots help support the bones and teeth, yes, teeth, of babies as they are developing.

CINNAMON: First, cinnamon makes anything tastes better. Adding a pinch of cinnamon to oatmeal or beverages can take something that is naturally bland and turn it into something rich and comforting. When it comes to pregnancy, cinnamon is great for women with gestational diabetes (that was me). Cinnamon not only helps regulate and promote healthy sugar absorption, but it can also help blood sugar levels for women with type 2 diabetes. Please be mindful about your cinnamon consumption, though, as large amounts of cinnamon could cause contractions.

GINGER: Ginger is a wonderful ingredient during pregnancy, especially in the first trimester. It can help with nausea, morning sickness, and vomiting. Although it is an acquired taste and strong, it can be a tremendous help when suffering from these symptoms. Another benefit of ginger is that it helps the body absorb more nutrients, which is beneficial for moms-to-be and their unborn babies. Between occasional lack of appetite and phases of crazy cravings, your body needs as much good stuff as possible.

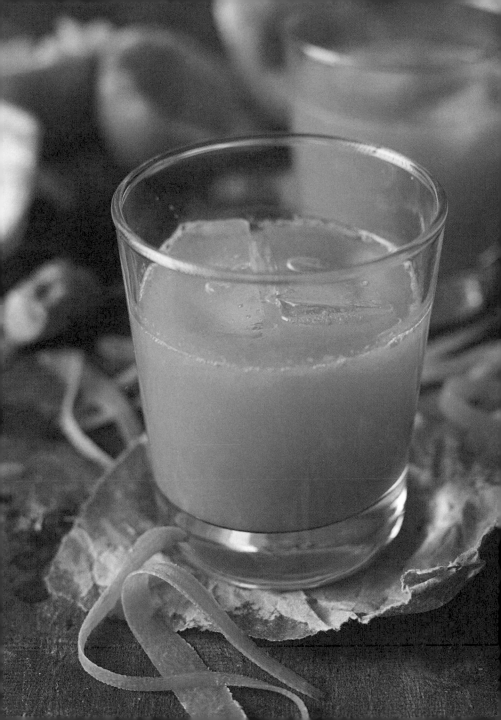

GRAPEFRUIT: Grapefruit is a great source of vitamin C, which is a huge immunity booster for you and your baby. Grapefruit also contains lycopene, a nutrient that helps lower blood pressure and can reduce the risk of preeclampsia.

HONEYDEW MELON: I am sure you wouldn't think honeydew melon has much ability to make an impact during pregnancy, but it does. In fact, due to its high water content, honeydew melon is a great way to stay hydrated, which is very important during pregnancy. Honeydew is high in potassium and it's great for the skin! You want to support that morning glow, don't you?

LEMONS: Lemons are a natural diuretic and have many health benefits for everyone, pregnant or not. Lemons are another natural ingredient that may help ward off morning sickness. In fact, eating lemons is a great way to get awesome vitamins and nutrients, such as vitamins C and B. They are also high in folic acid. Lemons naturally cleanse the liver and are another source of potassium, which is good for the heart!

MANGOES: Mangoes can help ease constipation and indigestion. Also, they are an energy booster. Believe me, you are going to need your energy, especially in the first trimester. Mangoes are loaded with vitamin B_6, which is very important for the baby's brain development and nervous system.

MATCHA GREEN TEA: Matcha green tea has great antioxidant properties and gives me energy. It does contain caffeine, so try to limit yourself to one glass a day.

PEACHES: One of my favorite fruits, especially in the summer when they are in season. Peaches are a natural detox agent. Of course, they contain vitamin C galore, which helps cleanse the liver and intestines of bad toxins and waste. Lastly, because peaches have a high fiber content, they can help ease constipation.

RED RASPBERRY LEAF TEA/PREGNANCY TEA: This tea is great for all sorts of pregnancy symptoms. It helps with morning sickness and relaxes the uterus to ease the pain and discomfort of childbirth. This tea can also help with breast milk supply and strengthening the mother's immune system. Along with these benefits, red raspberry leaf tea is said to decrease the chance of a miscarriage, and helps regulate postpartum hormones.

RHUBARB: This red-tinged celery look-alike is great for hypertension. Pregnancy with levels of hypertension can be dangerous, as it can lead to preeclampsia. Preeclampsia can put the mom at risk of serious brain injuries, liver and kidney malfunction, and seizures, and it can cause infant death. Rhubarb can help prevent hypertension; however, please always consult with your doctor if you are having severe symptoms related to this condition. It is also important to use only the stalks and to not eat the leaves of rhubarb, as the leaves can be poisonous.

TEA: The teas that you will see in these recipes not only serve as an alcohol replacement, but also add nutritional value that could provide some relief to some of the icky symptoms you may be feeling, such as nausea, fatigue, upset stomach, and headaches. For most of the recipes that require tea, I used two tea bags and heavily steeped the tea so the flavor could come through and I would get as much out of them as I could. You can use whatever brand of tea you want. To reap the most benefits, use loose leaf tea, as tea from less processed herbs can taste better and have more nutritional value.

SIMPLE SYRUP RECIPES

YIELD: About 1 cup syrup

To make these syrups, place the water, sweetener, and spice or herb in a medium saucepan. Bring to a boil and heat until the sugar has dissolved. Allow to cool before using and store in an airtight container. I use mason jars.

Basic Simple Syrup

1 cup water
1 cup sugar

Basil Simple Syrup

1 cup water
1 cup sugar
1 stem of basil

- -

Cinnamon Simple Syrup

1 cup water
1 cup sugar
1 teaspoon ground cinnamon
1 cinnamon stick

- -

Honey Simple Syrup

1 cup water
1 cup honey

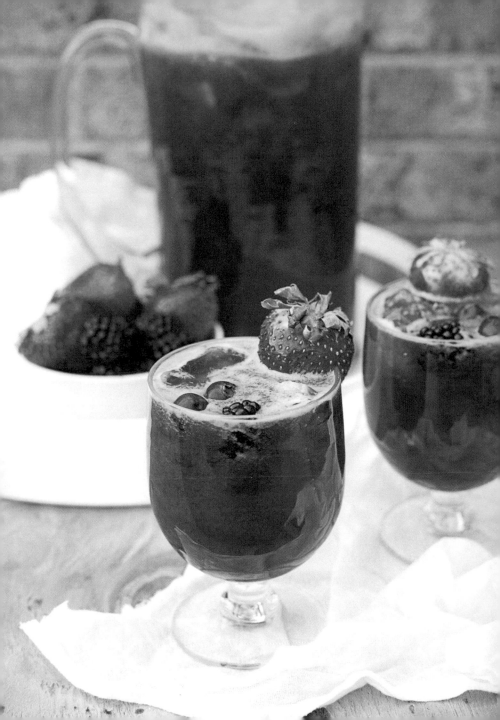

CHAPTER 1:

FROM the GARDEN

The First Trimester

YAY, YOU! YOU'RE PREGNANT AND LIFE IS GREAT! You and your significant other couldn't be more ecstatic about the little life that is growing inside you. You are thinking of all the things he or she could be. OMG! Is it a she or a he? What will you name your baby? What about your birthing plan? Will you go natural, water birth, or get an epidural? Will you have a coed baby shower or the traditional all-female shower with cute little finger sandwiches? What kind of mom will you be? Are you ready to be a mom? Will you breast- or bottle feed? I think you get the point. You have a lot going on in that beautiful mind of yours. It is enough to make you want a *drink*!

Ahh, a nice buzzy alcoholic beverage would take the edge off right about now. It most certainly will help you relax, with all that you have going and what you are thinking, right? *Wrong!* You are on a nine-month alcohol hiatus, my friend. Every emotion and thought you encounter from this point forward must be felt 100 percent sober. For some that is okay, but if you are anything like me, having a nice cocktail full of vodka, rum, and gin would be a nice way to soothe the morning sickness, the fatigue, the sore boobs, and the rainbow of emotions.

Cheer up, my friend! This section of mocktails will help support your health and provide some relief to those symptoms you are experiencing as you enjoy thinking about the life that is growing inside you.

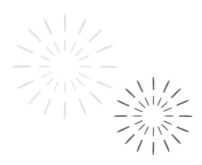

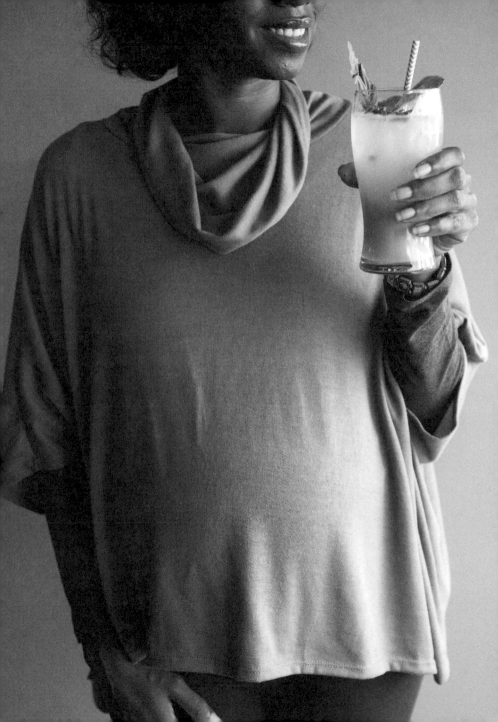

First Trimester Checklist

 SCHEDULE DOCTOR'S APPOINTMENT. You took a home pregnancy test; now it's time to get your pregnancy confirmed by your doctor. Schedule an appointment right now. Your regular health-care practitioner is fine for this step.

 SELECT YOUR OB-GYN. Start researching and interviewing OB-GYNs who may deliver your baby. Be sure to ask them questions about their policy for natural and C-section delivery, postnatal care, and patient expectations. Also, discuss any previous surgeries or pregnancy complications so your doctor can provide the best support and advice to ensure a happy and safe pregnancy.

 RESEARCH HOSPITAL FACILITIES. This was a big one for me. It was important that I toured the hospital, researched its labor and delivery rating and service, and got a sense of the overall staff support and comfort of the facility. I recommend that you ask your chosen doctor where he or she delivers so you can begin your research.

GET PRENATAL VITAMINS. These are essential, as they provide you and your baby the extra nutrients and vitamins that you both need during this time. Select prenatal vitamins that not only have positive nutritional properties but also provide nutrients that will support your baby's brain and spinal cord development.

 REVIEW HEALTH-CARE BENEFITS, DEDUCTIBLES, AND COVERAGE. It is important you know how much and what your health insurance will cover and what you will be left to pay for. Once you have these details, I recommend starting a savings account where you put aside a certain amount to pay for the medical bills you will incur once your baby is born.

 REFRAIN FROM SMOKING AND FROM DRINKING ALCOHOL. Well, that is why you bought this book!

CHANGE YOUR DIET. Raw meat, fish, undercooked eggs, and even certain cheeses can be unsafe to consume during pregnancy, as they contain bacteria (and in fish, mercury) that could be harmful to you and your baby. Don't eat them! Check with your doctor for a full list of potentially harmful foods and compensate by eating more good stuff, such as grains, fruits, vegetables, and legumes, for a healthy and sensible diet.

DRINK MORE WATER. I was crazy thirsty during my pregnancy. Be sure to drink plenty of water, especially if you live in a warm climate, as your body and baby need the extra fluid. Drinking plenty of water can prevent dehydration, which can cause nausea, dizziness, and cramps.

SHARE THE NEWS WITH YOUR FAMILY AND FRIENDS.
Be sure to surround yourself with family and friends who
will support and comfort you during this season in your life.
Let people know what you need, such as a meal, someone to do
laundry, a friend to watch *Sex and the City* with, or someone
to make you a mocktail from this book. Whatever you need,
be sure to surround yourself with people who you know will be
there for you.

- -

**REVIEW YOUR EMPLOYER'S MATERNITY LEAVE
POLICY AND SPEAK TO YOUR HR REP ABOUT YOUR
OPTIONS.** It is important that you know how much paid and
unpaid time you are allotted through your employer's terms
and policies. If you have a significant other, it is important,
too, for your partner to understand the amount of time his or
her job allows off so you can begin to plan to have as much time
with your baby postdelivery.

- -

Pear and Ginger Spritzer

YIELD: **2 servings**

This is an amazing drink to help soothe an upset tummy due to morning sickness and the discomfort due to constipation, and to awaken your taste buds due to the bland foods you're probably eating because food just doesn't sound that great to you right now. Not to worry; we have all been there. Although nothing sounds appetizing to you right now, I am sure this Pear and Ginger Spritzer will help to ease some of those first trimester symptoms so you can enjoy food again. Hang in there!

INGREDIENTS

4 Bartlett pears, or 2 cups pear nectar

One 1-inch piece fresh ginger

Ginger ale

GARNISH IDEAS
thin pear slices and fresh mint leaves

DIRECTIONS

Cut the pears, if using, into large chunks. Place the pears and ginger together in a juicer and juice per the manufacturer's instructions. Once the foam has settled, remove the foam by using a slotted or mesh spoon or other preferred method, leaving mostly juice. If using prepared juice, finely mince the ginger and divide between two glasses filled halfway with ice. Pour the pear juice into the ice-filled glasses and top off with ginger ale.

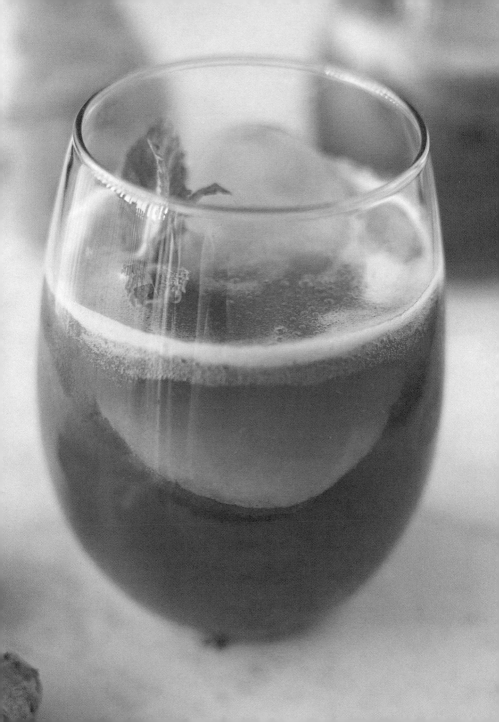

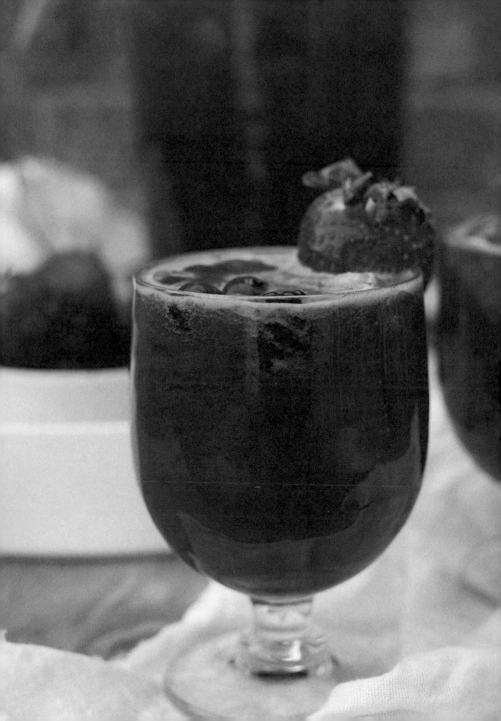

Mixed Berry Sangria

YIELD: **4 to 6 servings**

On a nice cool day, there is nothing better than a cool glass of sangria—red wine, delicious fruit, and a little fizz from some carbonated beverage. Well, I can't help you with the red wine, but I have replaced the wine with the red raspberry leaf tea (pregnancy tea) and a generous mix of the juice from mixed berries. If you don't have a juicer, try using a 100 percent–fruit fruit punch instead of the berries.

INGREDIENTS

4 cups water

2 red raspberry leaf tea bags

1 pound strawberries

6 ounces blueberries

6 ounces blackberries, plus extra for garnish

¼ cup Simple Syrup (page 22)

> GARNISH IDEA
> strawberry on the rim

DIRECTIONS

Brew the tea in 4 cups of water. You will need strong tea for this recipe. Hull the strawberries. Place half the strawberries and all the blueberries and blackberries in a juicer and juice per the manufacturer's instructions. Remove the foam, if desired. Fill a tall pitcher one-third of the way with ice. Pour the berry juice into the pitcher along with the tea, stir in the simple syrup, and add the remaining strawberries. Pour into your desired glasses.

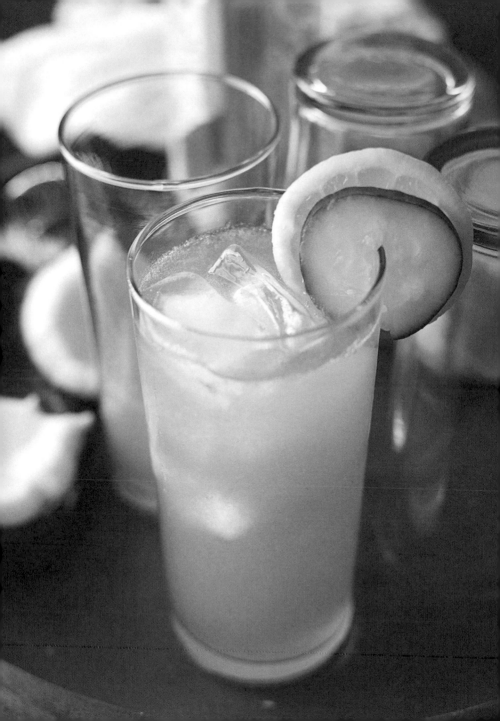

Fountain *of* Youth

YIELD: **2 servings**

This mocktail is full of ingredients that are not only good for you, but will help support that beautiful morning glow. Aloe vera juice is a great moisturizer, and the coconut water is good for aging. Not to mention that this drink is downright good! Drinking these two beverages separately may not be the best-tasting beverage there is, but together they are delicious and can add years to your appearance and radiance—not that you need it.

INGREDIENTS
½ cucumber
1 cup aloe vera juice
1 cup coconut water
Juice of 1 lemon
¼ cup Simple Syrup (page 22)

GARNISH IDEAS
cucumber and lemon slices

DIRECTIONS

Cut the cucumber into small pieces. Place the cucumber pieces in the middle of a piece of cheesecloth set over a large glass measuring cup. Squeeze the liquid from the cucumber several times until most of it is extracted, then discard the spent pulp. Alternately, muddle the cucumber with a wooden spoon. Add the aloe vera juice, coconut water, lemon juice, and simple syrup and stir. Serve in two large glasses filled with ice.

Asian-Inspired Hot Toddy

YIELD: **1 to 2 servings**

There are going to be days where you are not going to want to get out of bed. You are going to feel sick, uninspired, lazy, and downright crappy. Let me assure you, this too shall pass. But while you are lying in your bed eating saltine crackers and drinking your ginger ale, let me offer another alternative. Hot toddies are typically made with bourbon or whiskey, and seeing how you cannot have that, I want you to try this hot toddy that tastes like fruit and licorice. The goji berries, considered a superfood, are full of antioxidants, vitamins, and minerals that your body will love. The lemon, honey, star anise, and cinnamon are going to make you feel all warm and cozy inside.

INGREDIENTS

2 cups water

2 star anise

1 cinnamon stick

1 lemon slice

2 tablespoons goji berries

1½ tablespoons honey

2 teaspoons chopped fresh ginger

1 teaspoon bourbon flavoring

DIRECTIONS

Combine the water, star anise, cinnamon stick, lemon slice, goji berries, honey, and ginger in a medium saucepan and bring to a boil. Allow to steep for 10 minutes. Add the bourbon flavoring, stir, and pour into your desired coffee mug.

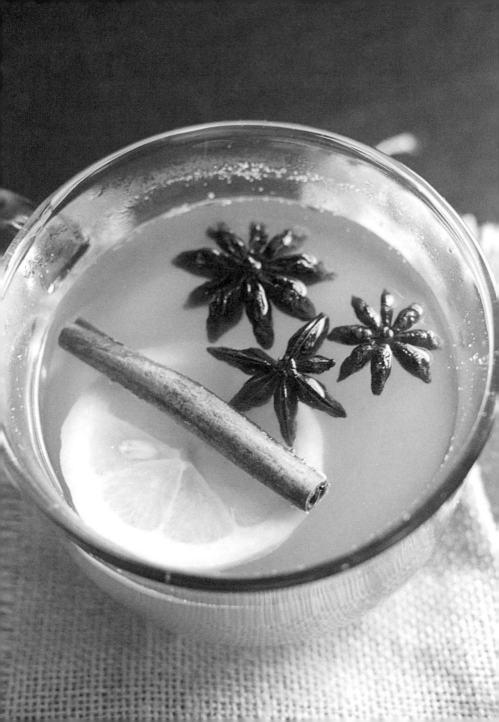

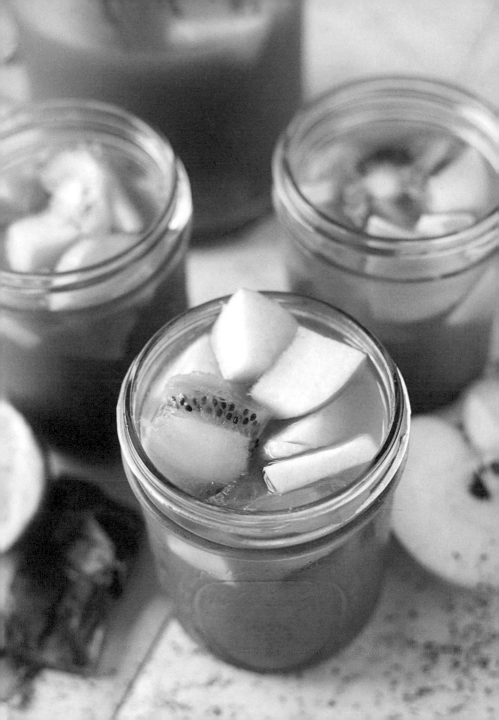

Mean Green Sangria

YIELD: **6 to 8 servings**

I know, I know. You're tired of people telling you how important it
is for you to be healthy. If you're anything like me, I *know* you are
tired of hearing all the advice about what to do and what not to do,
what to eat, what not to eat, and how to feed your child once he or
she arrives. It all can be very taxing and annoying. Well, as much
as I understand where you are right now, I am going to join that
group of people who are getting on your nerves and tell you to try
this superfood sangria. Mostly for one reason and one reason only.
Kombucha! I won't lie: kombucha is an acquired flavor that tastes
somewhat like vinegar. But really, it isn't that bad. In fact, I love
it. Kombucha is referred to as the elixir of life! Why wouldn't you
want that goodness in your body?!

INGREDIENTS

4 cups water

2 green tea bags

1 bunch kale

8 ounces fresh spinach

5 green apples: 3 cut into chunks, 2 cored and sliced (reserve for serving)

4 kiwis, peeled: 2 chopped, 2 sliced (reserve for serving)

1 cucumber, cut into chunks

Juice of 1 lime

3 ounces Simple Syrup (page 22)

8 ounces kombucha

continued

DIRECTIONS

Brew the tea in 4 cups of water. You will need strong tea for this recipe. Place the kale, spinach, apple chunks, chopped kiwi, and cucumber chunks in a juicer and juice per the manufacturer's instructions. Once the juice has settled, use a slotted or mesh spoon to remove the foam. Fill a pitcher one-third of the way with ice. Pour in the juice and the tea. Stir in the lime juice and simple syrup. Add the apple and kiwi slices, top off with the kombucha, and serve.

NOTE: If you don't have a juicer, substitute 3 cups of your favorite green juice for the kale, spinach, 3 apples, 2 kiwis, and cucumber.

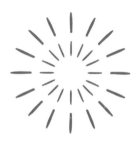

"Morning Sickness Fixer" Ginger Fizz

YIELD: 2 to 3 servings

So, I had the worst kind of morning sickness when I was pregnant with my baby. I was lightheaded, dizzy, nauseous, and just felt sick all the time. I tried the saltine cracker and ginger ale concoction, I tried "preggy pops," and I even drank chicken and beef broth. Although these remedies did help some, there was nothing that completely cured these symptoms. The good news is if you are experiencing these symptoms, it means your baby is off to a healthy start. If that isn't enough for you, try this mocktail I like to call the "Morning Sickness Fixer." It is full of ginger and a hint of lemon. It may not cure all your symptoms completely, but it can provide some relief. Hang in there, momma.

INGREDIENTS

4 cups water
2 ginger tea bags
1 tablespoon chopped fresh ginger
2 tablespoons honey
Ginger beer

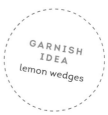

GARNISH IDEA
lemon wedges

DIRECTIONS

Brew the tea in 4 cups of water. You will need strong tea for this recipe. For each serving, fill an 8-ounce glass halfway with ice, pour in some of the tea, and top off with some of the ginger beer.

Mixed Berry Hibiscus Spritzer

YIELD: **2 to 4 servings**

I found a delicious hibiscus fruity tea and I just had to try it. You are going to see a lot of berries in this book, as I just love them! Not to mention, berries are great to eat during your pregnancy. With the right flavors, you will appreciate berries in a whole new way!

INGREDIENTS

4 cups water

1 hibiscus berry tea bag

Mixed berries (strawberries, blackberries, and raspberries)

Berry-flavored carbonated water

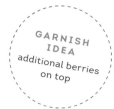

GARNISH IDEA
additional berries on top

DIRECTIONS

Brew the tea in 4 cups of water. You will need strong tea for this recipe. Place a couple of mixed berries in the bottom of two to four glasses. Muddle the berries just enough to release the berry juices. Add some ice on top and pour in the tea to fill halfway. Finish by adding the berry-carbonated water the rest of the way.

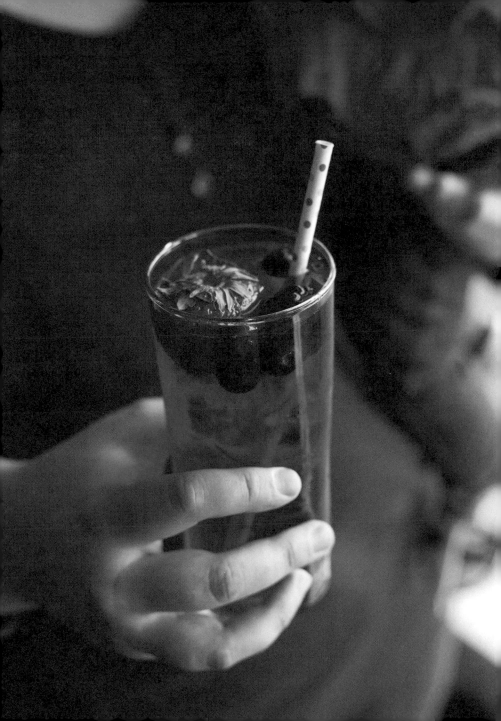

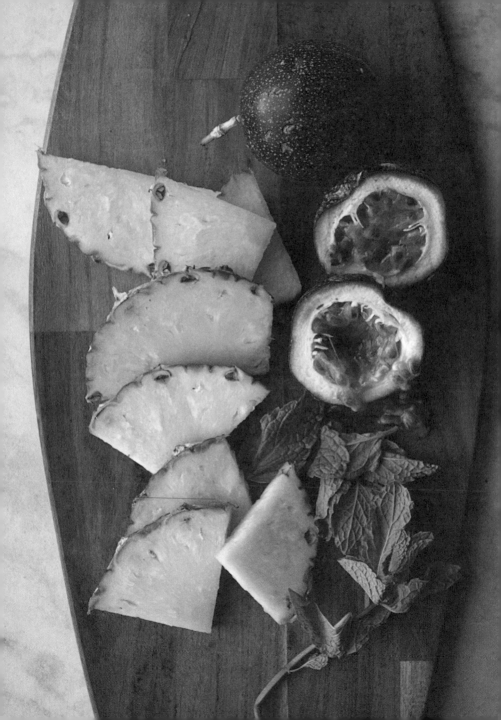

Passion Fruit and Mint Mojito

YIELD: **1 serving**

I absolutely, positively *love* passion fruit. When my husband and I were on our honeymoon, I ate passion fruit every day for breakfast. Imagine my delight when I found passion fruit being sold at a local market. I had to put passion fruit in a drink or two! Sure, I could've used passion fruit syrup only, but there is nothing like the real thing. I had to make this drink so you guys can see what heaven tastes like.

INGREDIENTS

1 sprig of mint
1 whole passion fruit
2 ounces passion fruit syrup
½ teaspoon rum flavoring
3 ounces pineapple juice
2 ounces club soda

GARNISH
IDEA
pineapple wedge

DIRECTIONS

Place the mint in a large drinking glass and use a muddler or the back of a spoon to break up the leaves. Place the insides of the passion fruit, plus the passion fruit syrup, rum flavoring, and pineapple juice in a shaker. Shake hard for about 1 minute and strain the drink into the drinking glass, allowing some of the passion fruit seeds into the glass. Place the lid from the shaker on top of the drinking glass and shake a couple of times to allow everything to mix with the mint. Top with club soda.

Cucumber Lemonade

The first time I had cucumber lemonade was at a restaurant where I wanted to try something new, something different. No kidding, when I took my first sip of this amazing lemonade concoction, my eyes lit up and I said, "Well, hot darn!" I love the refreshing flavor that came from the cucumber and the mint, and the tartness that came from the lemons. It was the perfect combination for a refreshing beverage. I hope you find it to be the same.

INGREDIENTS

12 large lemons

3 cucumbers

2 sprigs of mint

1 cup Simple Syrup (page 22)

8 cups water

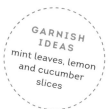

GARNISH IDEAS
mint leaves, lemon and cucumber slices

DIRECTIONS

Using a citrus juicer, juice 10 of the lemons. Slice two of the cucumbers in half and then dice. Place the diced cucumber in the middle of a piece of cheesecloth set over a large glass measuring cup. Squeeze the liquid from the cucumber several times until most of it is extracted, then discard the spent pulp. Place the lemon juice, cucumber juice, mint sprigs, simple syrup, and water in a gallon-size pitcher. Slice the remaining two lemons and the remaining cucumber and add the slices to the pitcher. Serve over ice.

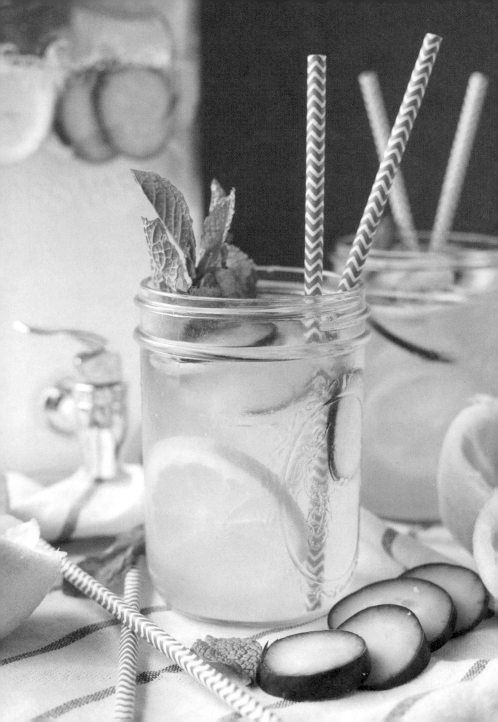

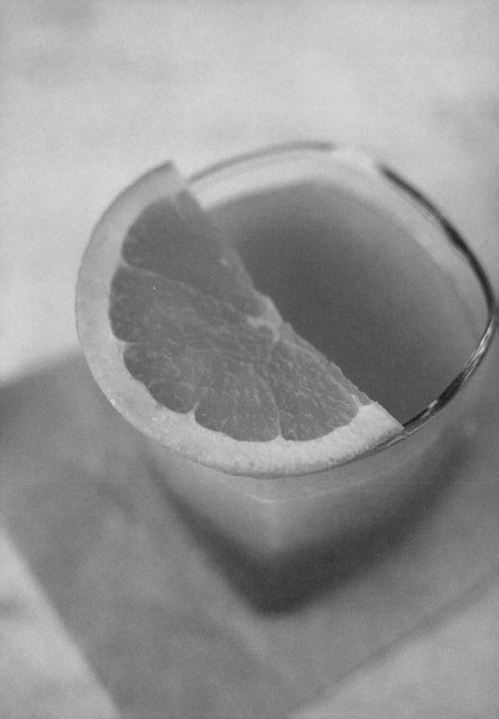

Baby Sunrise

YIELD: **1 serving**

How awesome this would taste with tequila—I can see why they call it a Tequila Sunrise. Well, this recipe still makes for a great mocktail . . . just without the tequila. Here, we are using freshly squeezed orange juice and a shot of grenadine. That's it! So simple yet so delicious.

INGREDIENTS
Juice of 4 large navel oranges
1 ounce grenadine

DIRECTIONS
Pour the orange juice into a snifter glass, then pour in the grenadine.

GARNISH IDEAS
maraschino cherries and ½ orange slice

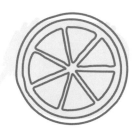

Cinnamon Apple-Tini

YIELD: **1 to 2 servings**

If you're anything like me, you love yourself one sweet, tart, and strong apple martini. If only you could have an apple martini right now, right? Well, this variation will still do the trick.

INGREDIENTS

10 ounces fresh apple juice
   (from about 4 large Fuji or Honeycrisp apples)
5 ounces heavily brewed chai tea
1 ounce Cinnamon Simple Syrup (page 23)
1 teaspoon bourbon flavoring
1 lemon wedge
Cinnamon sugar, for rim

GARNISH IDEAS
slice of apple and sugared rim (see note, page 77)

DIRECTIONS

Once you have juiced the apples, remove the foam with a slotted or mesh spoon. Pour the apple juice, chai tea, cinnamon simple syrup, and bourbon flavoring into a shaker and squeeze in the juice from the lemon wedge. Shake well and pour in a cinnamon sugar-rimmed martini glass.

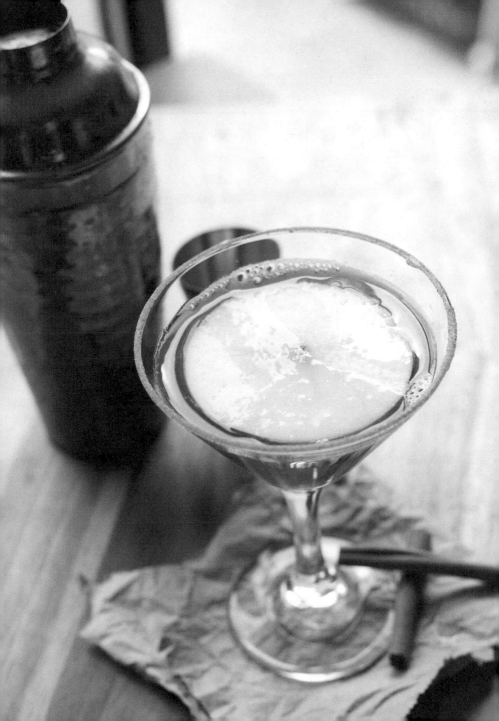

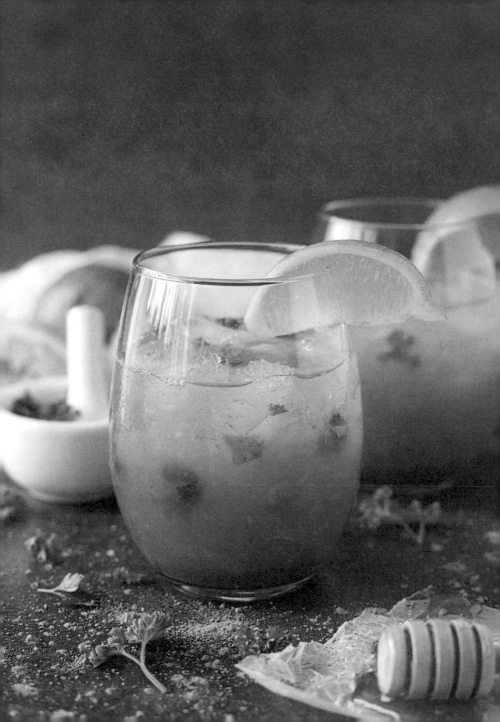

Matcha, Honey, and Lime, Oh My!

YIELD: 2 to 3 servings

I prefer matcha green tea over leaf green tea any day. You see, I am not much of a coffee person. Don't get me wrong; I love some aspects of coffee, but I prefer to get my caffeine through my matcha tea. Not only do I love to have my matcha tea hot, but this lovely mocktail makes me appreciate having it chilled as well. This is a delicious beverage that I could enjoy on a hot day when I need a pick-me-up.

INGREDIENTS

4 cups water
1 tablespoon matcha green tea powder
5 sprigs of parsley
2 ounces Honey Simple Syrup (page 23)
Juice from ½ lime
Juice from ½ lemon

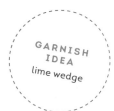

GARNISH IDEA
lime wedge

DIRECTIONS

Bring the water to a boil in a saucepan, remove from the heat, and add the matcha powder. Use a whisk to blend the matcha into the water. Allow the tea to cool. Using a mortar and pestle, muddle the parsley, add it to the green tea, and whisk. Add the honey simple syrup and the lime and lemon juice. Pour over ice.

Orange and Turmeric Elixir

Okay, so do I need to say that turmeric is amazing? If so, turmeric is amazing! This, too, has many anti-inflammatory properties that can help with pain and swelling. It is superloaded with antioxidants and great for your liver! This elixir is a great way to get some vital nutrients in your body that you and that growing baby both can appreciate.

INGREDIENTS

2½ ounces fresh turmeric or 1½ teaspoons turmeric powder
2 carrots
Juice of 4 navel oranges
Splash of tonic water

DIRECTIONS

Place the fresh turmeric, if using, and carrots in a juicer and juice per the manufacturer's instructions. Mix the orange juice and carrot mixture together in a large shaker, and add the turmeric powder, if using. Pour into four 8-ounce glasses filled with ice, pour a splash of tonic water on top, and serve.

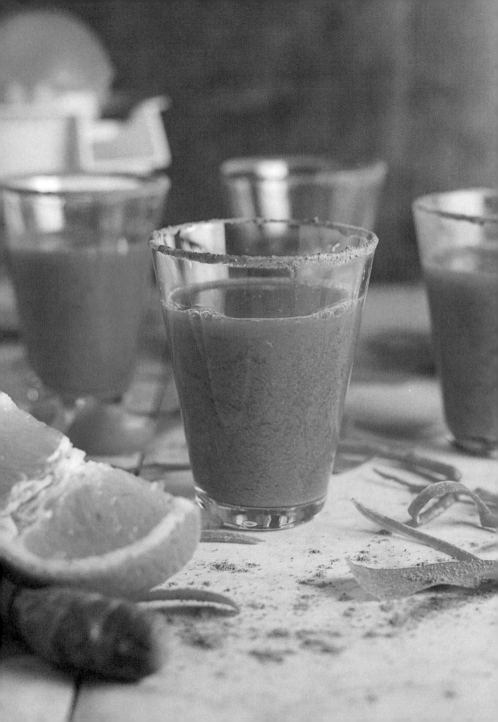

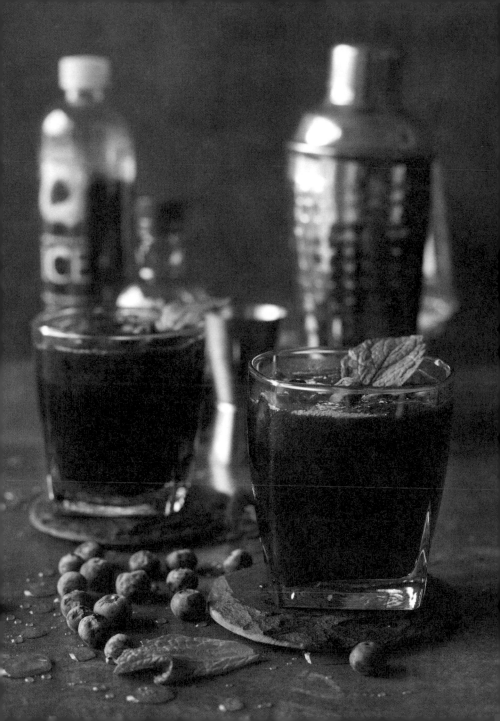

Momma Baby Blues Mocktail

YIELD: **1 serving**

There is another superhero among the berries. I am talking pure pomegranate juice! Have you ever seen that pomegranate commercial where the juice acts like an army or fight squad against that bad stuff in your body? Well, even if you haven't seen it, that is exactly what pomegranate juice does. It is a great asset to your body's defense system against free radicals and unwanted stuff that could make you sick or feel sluggish. So, if you have the blues, just make this mocktail and let the good stuff in this drink do the rest.

INGREDIENTS

12 ounces blueberries
6 ounces blackberries
8 ounces pomegranate juice
Blueberry-flavored carbonated water

GARNISH IDEAS
mint leaves and blueberries

DIRECTIONS

Place the berries and juice in a blender and puree. Fill a small glass with ice, strain in the juice mixture to about two-thirds of the way full, and top off with the berry-flavored carbonated water.

Green Grape and Basil Spritzer

YIELD: **2 to 4 servings**

I am a sucker for grapes. Especially sweet, plump, and slightly sour green grapes. Oh my goodness, they are *everything*! I know they are fruit and all, but I call them "earth candy" because they are so sweet and delicious. It doesn't feel as if I'm eating something healthy. If you feel the same way, then this mocktail is going to be nothing short of delicious.

INGREDIENTS

1 pound green grapes
1.5 ounces Basil Simple Syrup (page 23)
One 25.4-ounce bottle nonalcoholic sparkling wine

DIRECTIONS

Place the grapes and syrup in a blender and puree. Fill two to four glasses halfway with ice, strain in the juice mixture to about two-thirds of the way full, and top off with the grape sparkling wine.

GARNISH IDEAS
frozen green grapes and fresh basil leaves

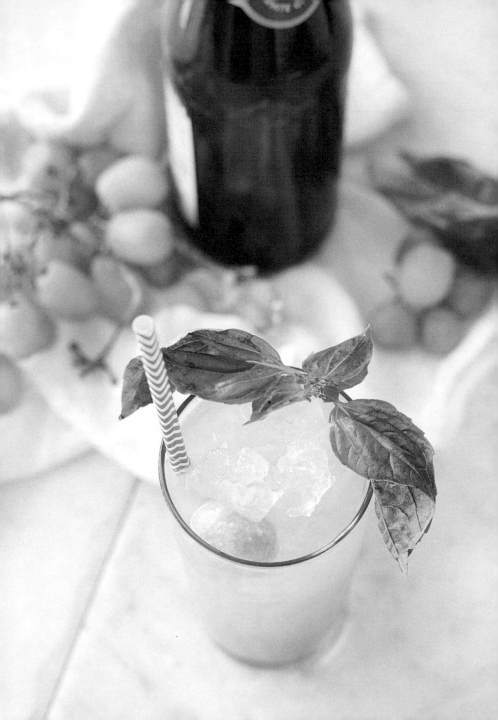

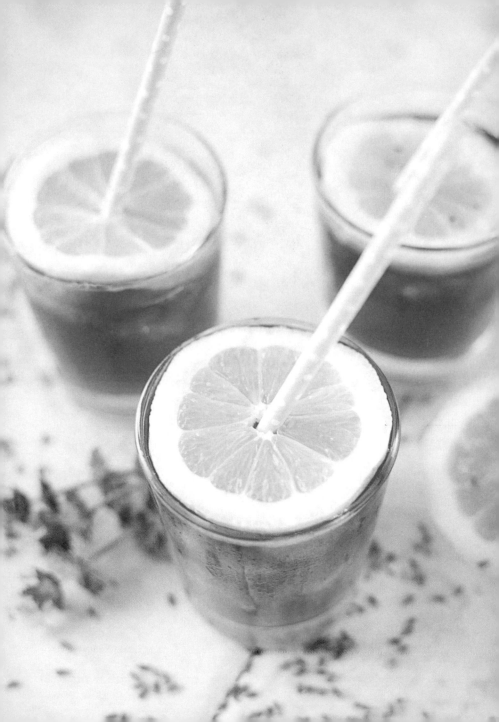

Lavender Lemonade

Lavender is absolutely my most favorite flower. Oh, I love the way it smells and looks. The color is so gorgeous to me. True story: Once I saw a bush of lavender growing in the city while I was driving and I pulled over and took a large bundle of lavender to keep in my house. Sure, I looked like a crazy lavender lady, but I had to have it! I even have sachets of lavender buds in my dresser drawers. Soooo, it only makes sense that I find a way to consume the delicate flower. This drink is perfect and will bring out the lavender lover in anyone.

INGREDIENTS

3 cups water
1½ tablespoons dried culinary-grade lavender buds
Juice of 3 large lemons
¼ cup Simple Syrup (page 22)
Food coloring (optional)

DIRECTIONS

Bring the water to a boil in a saucepan and add the lavender buds. Boil for 5 to 10 minutes, then remove from the heat and allow to cool. In a small pitcher, combine lavender tea, lemon juice, and simple syrup. Pour into two or three 8-ounce glasses filled with ice. Use food coloring, if desired, to bring out the lavender color.

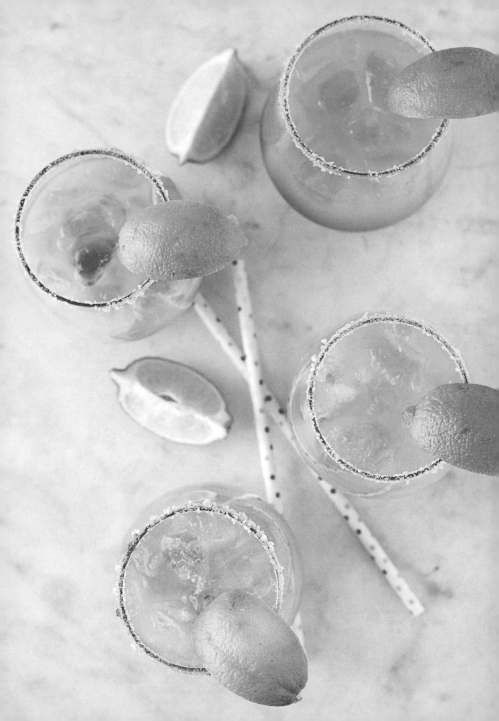

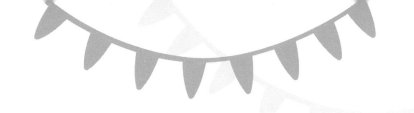

CHAPTER 2:

BOOZE-FREE CLASSICS

The Second Trimester

ALL RIGHT, YOU HAVE MADE IT OUT OF THE DARK AGES!
Well, at least I hope so. Now you are starting to feel like your
normal self and doing things you used to do. You probably got
your appetite back as well. I remember eating anything and
everything during my second trimester until I found out I had
gestational diabetes and had to go on a strict diet, which I don't
wish on anyone. If that is not an issue for you, enjoy yourself.
Still eat healthy, though. Some things you can expect during this
phase: seeing your belly round out, starting to think about your
baby shower and about buying maternity clothes, and, finally, if
you're going to find out the sex of your baby. *Yay!* Or not. Whatever
you decide, just enjoy these three months because one more
uncomfortable phase follows. Just thought I'd break that to you
before you get too excited.

Second Trimester Checklist

 BEGIN PLANNING YOUR BABY SHOWER. I don't know about you, but this made my pregnancy! We had the best baby shower our family and friends have ever seen! I didn't want a traditional all-female baby shower. I wanted my husband to be included and a part of every aspect of my pregnancy, which moved us to have a coed baby shower. Because we are a huge football family, it only made sense to throw a tailgate party dressed as a baby shower. It was super fun! I encourage you to work with your significant other to determine how involved he or she will want to be in planning this event and come up with something that will work for both of you.

 START DECORATING YOUR NURSERY. Once you find out the sex of your baby, it is time to pick a nursery theme! This is where Pinterest will become your best friend and your new addiction. I think I was on Pinterest all day, every day. Look around for the best possible deals to decorate the room for your little one and find some DIY projects that are easy and safe for you to do, as it can give you and your significant other more time to talk and bond before the baby arrives.

DO YOUR RESEARCH. I took an online class that teaches a safe and effective sleeping schedule for babies, one that helps them sleep well starting at a young age. Unfortunately, I found out about this class when my baby was no longer considered a newborn but an infant. However, I still followed the steps and he is still on that same sleeping schedule, and it did help him learn to sleep well at night. I can't help but wonder, though, had I found out about that class earlier, whether I would've had more nights with more rest. I am telling you from my own experience to start looking up sleep schedules, information about vaccinations, and tips on breast- versus bottle-feeding now, so when your baby arrives you have some structure and sense of direction of things you want to do with your baby.

PLAN YOUR BIRTHING PLAN. You should be talking more about your options for delivery and learning what to expect based upon your decision. I had to have a C-section, so I asked a lot of questions about the procedure: what I could expect before, during, and after the surgery; about recovery; and, because I'm a punk, what kind of pain relief options I would have. I recommend that you schedule this conversation close to the end of your second trimester and come with a list of questions to ask your health-care provider.

PLAN A "BABYMOON" AND REMEMBER THAT FEELING. A "babymoon" is something we New Age moms came up with, kind of like a honeymoon before the baby arrives. You and your significant other are going to go through many changes and challenges. If this is your first child, adding another person to your day-to-day lives is great, but it can put a strain on the two of you. It is important that you both understand this going forward and commit to ways that the two of you will continue to be close.

I can say from my own experience that there was an adjustment period between my husband and me when I felt as though we didn't talk about anything but the baby for a while. We completely underestimated what was required for the both of us to stay connected. Luckily we have great parents and friends whom we trusted to watch our baby while we enjoyed time with each other.

CREATE A LIST OF BABYSITTERS AND DAYCARE PROVIDERS. I cannot tell you how much this is going to be an ongoing conversation, but it needs to happen. Write a list of family and friends whom you trust to watch your baby for date nights or other occasions. This is important because you need to create a list of people whom you not only trust to watch your baby, but who will support any schedule or coping mechanisms that you have in place. My baby's sleeping schedule at night was determined by how successful his schedule was during the day. Therefore, I needed my babysitters to understand that and to not push their ideas and agenda on my baby. Make sure you make this clear to anyone watching your baby. After all, you are going to be stuck picking up the pieces of what your child minder does or doesn't do while you're away.

Baby Momma *on the* Beach

YIELD: **1 serving**

What happens on the beach is how you got yourself in the situation you're in now. Now that you are going to be a momma, let's have a nice stroll on the beach while you enjoy your pregnancy, shall we?

INGREDIENTS

2 ounces nonalcoholic peach cocktail mix
2 ounces orange juice
1.5 ounces cranberry juice
1 ounce grenadine
Splash of lemon-lime soda

DIRECTIONS

Fill a shaker halfway with ice and add the peach mix, orange juice, and cranberry juice. Shake well for about 30 seconds. Fill an 8- to 10-ounce glass halfway with ice and pour the juice mixture over the ice. Pour in the grenadine, add a splash of lemon-lime soda, and serve.

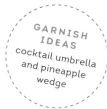

GARNISH IDEAS
cocktail umbrella and pineapple wedge

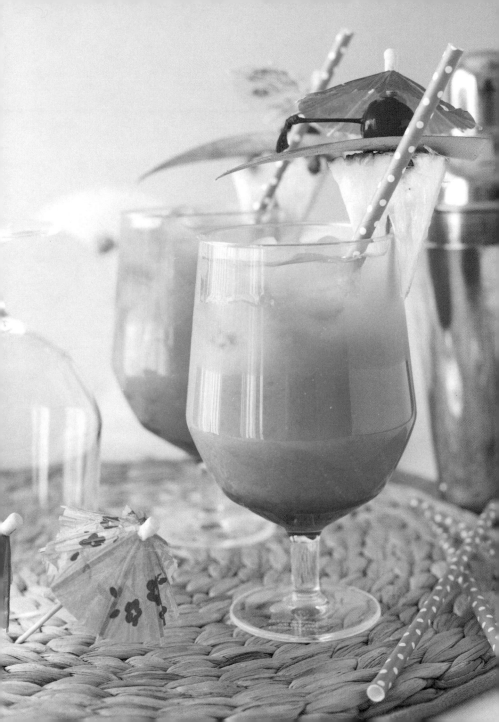

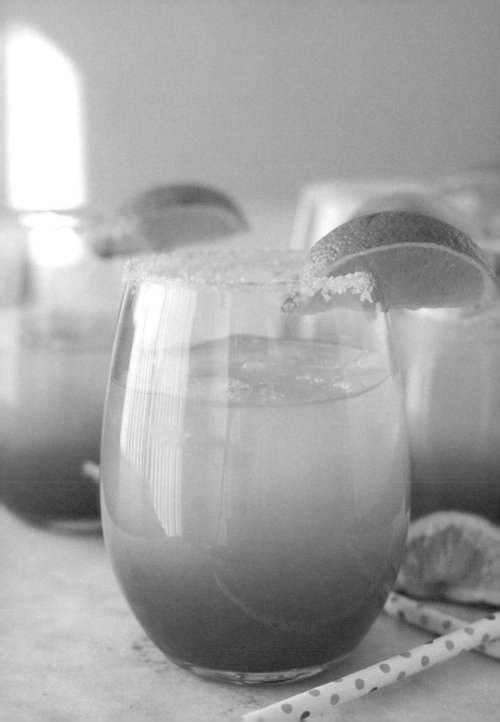

Mommy Tai

YIELD: 1 to 2 servings

Here is a mocktail version of another classic drink, the mai tai.
This delicious concoction of fruit juices does put you in the mind-
set of having a nice, relaxing drink at a wet bar at a beach resort. I
wish my husband and I could've had a drink like this at a wet bar at
a beach resort before our baby arrived. Thanks to Zika, we couldn't
travel to anywhere tropical. Oh well, this drink allows me to dream.

INGREDIENTS

2 ounces fresh orange juice
2 ounces fresh pineapple juice
Juice of 1 lime, squeezed
1 teaspoon rum flavoring
Splash of lemon-lime soda
Splash of grenadine

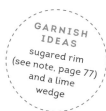

GARNISH IDEAS
sugared rim
(see note, page 77)
and a lime
wedge

DIRECTIONS

Fill a shaker halfway with ice, pour in the orange, pineapple, and lime
juices and rum flavoring, and shake. Pour into a glass filled halfway
with ice. Add a splash each of lemon-lime soda and grenadine.

Virgin Amaretto Sour

YIELD: 1 serving

Okay, this is one of my most favorite cocktails *ever*! It was the first cocktail I ever had that I fell in love with. So you can imagine my enthusiasm when I figured out how to make a virgin version of the Amaretto Sour. This classic cocktail can be enjoyed either with or without alcohol.

INGREDIENTS

2 ounces amaretto syrup

3 ounces Dr Pepper

2 ounces sweet-and-sour cocktail mix

DIRECTIONS

Fill a small glass half way with ice. Pour in the amaretto syrup, Dr Pepper, and sweet-and-sour cocktail mix.

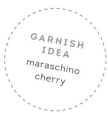

GARNISH IDEA
maraschino cherry

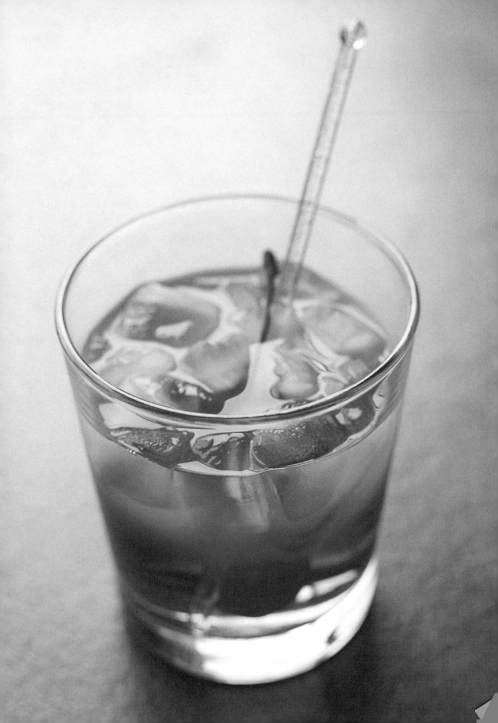

Cosmopolitan

YIELD: **1 serving**

I love *Sex and the City*! It would only be right as a fan to make this classic cocktail and share it with the rest of the world. Sure, it only has two ingredients without the alcohol, but that is what makes this mocktail so great. Remember, we are using juices that are freshly juiced or as pure as possible. Using pure cranberry juice and sweetened juice is what makes this mocktail a fan favorite.

INGREDIENTS
4 ounces pure cranberry juice
2 ounces sweetened lime juice

DIRECTIONS
Fill a shaker with ice and pour in the cranberry juice along with the lime juice. Shake to chill and pour into a martini glass.

NOTE: To sugar the rim of the martini glass, rub a lime wedge around the edge and dip the rim into a small dish of sugar. For a salted rim, swap out the sugar for salt.

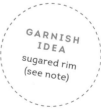

GARNISH
IDEA
sugared rim
(see note)

Virgin Piña Colada

YIELD: **4 servings**

"If you like piña coladas . . ." I don't know the rest of the song!
I have made a delicious creamy virgin piña colada that will have
you hearing the ocean waves in the background. Using real coconut
milk and pineapple, how could you go wrong?!

INGREDIENTS

6 cups frozen pineapple

1 cup nonalcoholic piña colada mix

½ cup pure coconut milk (not coconut milk
    beverage)

2 tablespoons coconut syrup

3 ounces pineapple juice

GARNISH
IDEAS
pineapple
wedge, coconut
shavings

DIRECTIONS

Place the still-frozen pineapple, piña colada mix, coconut milk,
coconut syrup, and pineapple juice in a blender. Blend on high
speed for 2 to 3 minutes, until smooth and creamy.

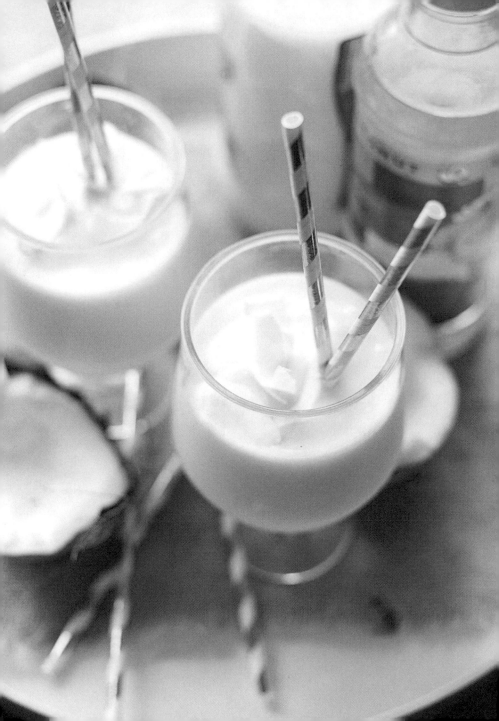

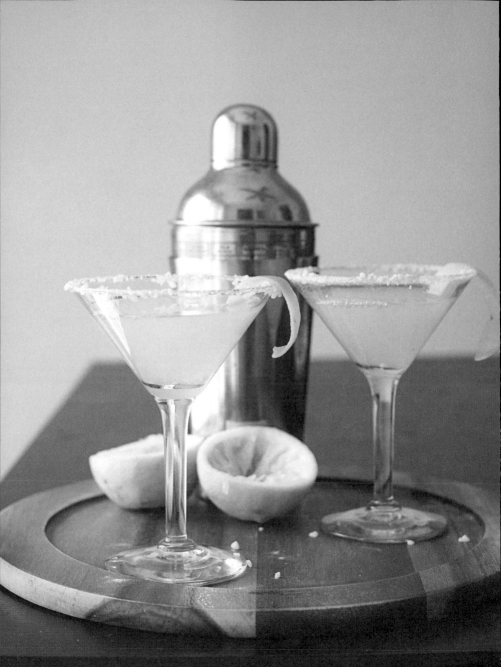

Lemon Drop Martini with Basil

YIELD: **2 servings**

This martini was not a part of my original plan. Initially, I was trying to go for something that tasted exactly like Lemonheads. You know, the candy? Well, that turned into a disaster, so this martini was a nice accident waiting to happen. Lemon and basil, what a beautiful marriage of flavors.

INGREDIENTS

Juice of 4 large lemons

2 fresh basil leaves

2 ounces Basil Simple Syrup (page 23)

DIRECTIONS

Fill a shaker halfway with ice. Pour in the lemon juice, add the basil leaves and basil simple syrup, and shake well. Pour into a martini glass.

GARNISH IDEA

crushed Lemonheads candy around the rim

Frozen Margarita

YIELD: **4 servings**

Here is another favorite of mine. The infamous margarita.
You will love this mocktail even without the tequila. Just bring
on the Mexican cuisine and you are in Cancún.

INGREDIENTS

Two 9-ounce nonalcoholic margarita mixers or limeade, frozen
1 cup nonalcoholic margarita mix
Juice of 1 lime

DIRECTIONS

Place the still-frozen margarita mixer or limeade, margarita mix,
and lime juice in a blender. Pulse on high speed until smooth.
Pour into four glasses.

GARNISH IDEAS
salted rim and lime wedge (see note, page 77)

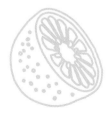

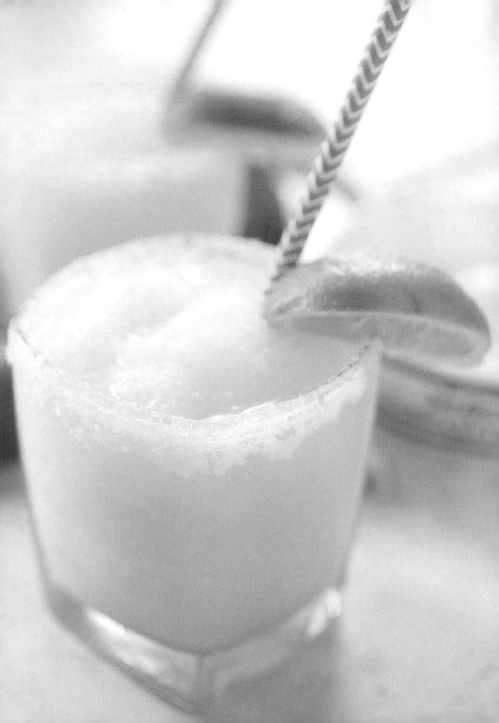

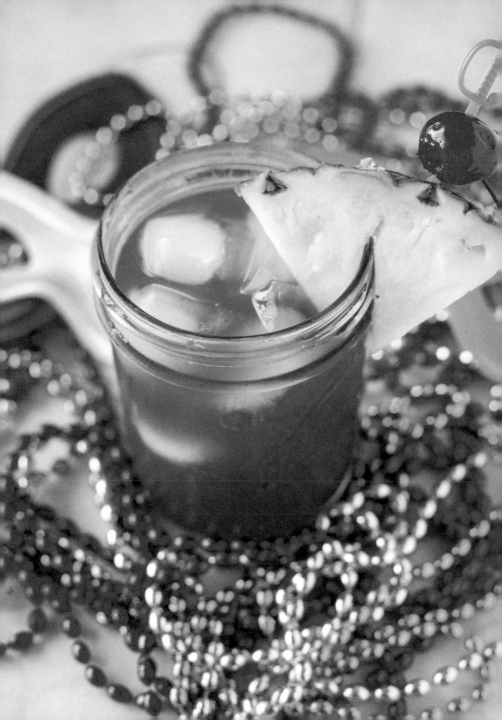

Hurricane

YIELD: 1 serving

Oh, how I love New Orleans. I go there just to eat, listen to music, and have a good Hurricane. You know you have a good Hurricane when you can't taste the alcohol, and that happens every time I am in New Orleans. All I taste is goodness and heaven. You will taste the same thing with this mocktail, and you'll swear there is real rum in it. I promise, there isn't.

INGREDIENTS

1 whole passion fruit

3 ounces orange juice

2 ounces cranberry juice

1 ounce grenadine

1 ounce lemon-lime soda

½ teaspoon rum flavoring

GARNISH IDEAS
cocktail umbrella, pineapple, and a maraschino cherry

DIRECTIONS

Fill a shaker halfway with ice. Cut the passion fruit in half, scoop out the insides of the fruit, and place in the shaker. Add the remaining ingredients, but not the lemon-lime soda. Shake vigorously to break apart the passion fruit. Fill a glass with ice and pour the drink into the glass while barely straining the fruit, allowing some of the passion fruit seeds into the drink. Pour in the lemon-lime soda and serve.

Grapefruit Pink Lady

YIELD: 1 to 2 servings

No, this cocktail does not contain bourbon, but it makes me think of women at the Kentucky Derby. I just imagine the women in their pretty dresses and large hats, drinking this beverage and talking about . . . whatever women who go to the Kentucky Derby talk about. I love this mocktail because it tastes pretty, if that makes any sense. The rose water just adds this nice, fragrant note to the drink that makes you feel like a lady. A Pink Lady, that is.

INGREDIENTS

Juice of 1 grapefruit or ½ cup pure grapefruit juice
Juice of 1 large navel orange or ⅓ cup pure orange juice
Juice of 1 lemon
1.5 ounces Honey Simple Syrup (page 23)
1.5 ounces rose water

DIRECTIONS

Fill a large shaker halfway with ice and add the grapefruit, orange, and lemon juice, honey simple syrup, and rose water. Shake well and pour in your desired cocktail glass(es).

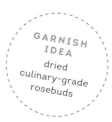

GARNISH IDEA
dried culinary-grade rosebuds

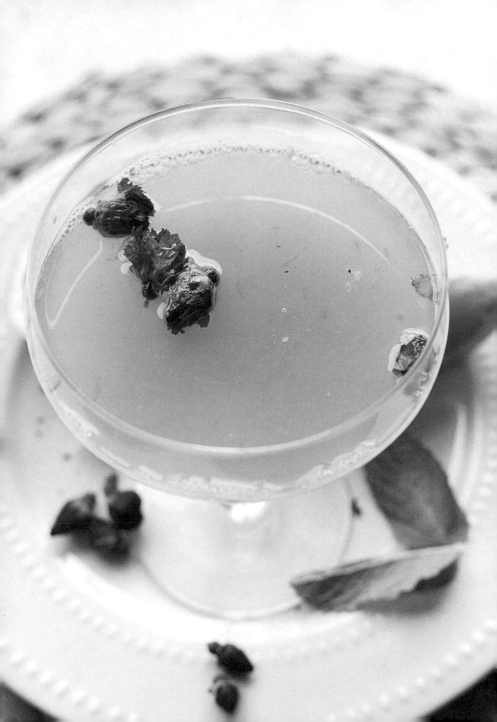

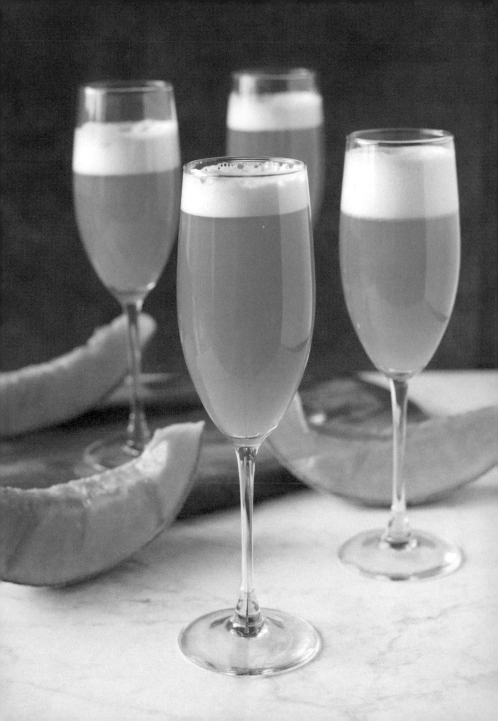

Cantaloupe Mimosa

Full disclosure: I am not a fan of cantaloupe. Never have been and I have tried. Wait a minute. I mean I don't like cantaloupe, the fruit, but I love cantaloupe juice. Especially in this mimosa. It is so refreshing and a wonderful alternative to the traditional mimosa.

INGREDIENTS
1½ pounds cantaloupe chunks
Melon-flavored carbonated water

DIRECTIONS
Place the cantaloupe in a juicer and juice per the manufacturer's instructions, then remove the foam with a slotted or mesh spoon. If you do not have a juicer, blend the cantaloupe pieces with ¼ cup of the carbonated water in a blender. Strain the juice and proceed with recipe. Pour the juice into four champagne flutes to fill halfway, then top off with melon-flavored carbonated water.

Strawberry Daiquiri

YIELD: **4 servings**

The Strawberry Daiquiri is a cocktail that anyone can love. Who wouldn't want a glass with delicious strawberries topped with whipped cream?!

INGREDIENTS

6 cups frozen strawberries

1 cup strawberry puree (such as Finest Call)

DIRECTIONS

Combine the still-frozen strawberries and strawberry puree in a blender and blend until smooth. Pour into your desired cocktail glasses.

GARNISH IDEAS
whipped cream and strawberries

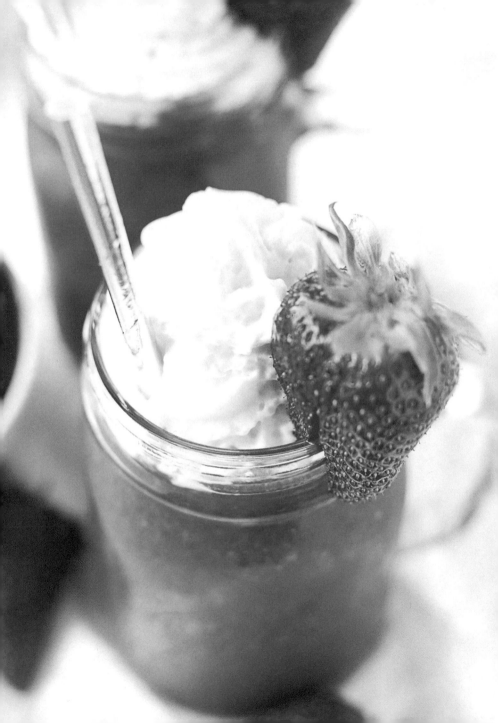

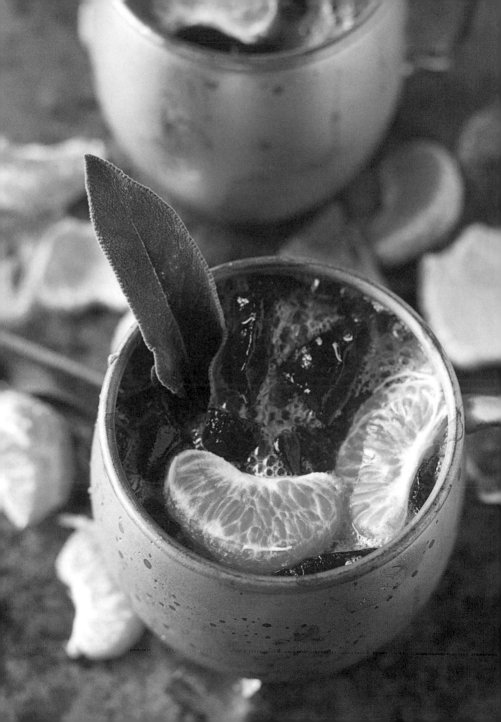

Clementine and Sage Moscow Mule

YIELD: **2 servings**

You will never believe how amazing the juice from a clementine and sage are together. Adding the ginger ale to these two flavors makes one fantastic Moscow Mule. I think the people of Moscow would love this mule.

INGREDIENTS
2 fresh sage leaves
Juice of 5 to 6 clementines
Ginger ale

DIRECTIONS

Muddle the two sage leaves. Fill a shaker with ice, add the sage and the clementine juice, and shake vigorously to release the flavor. Fill two copper mugs with ice. Pour the clementine juice equally between the mugs and top off with ginger ale.

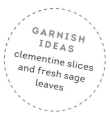

GARNISH IDEAS
clementine slices and fresh sage leaves

Blackberry Mojito

YIELD: **4 servings**

Blackberry. Lime. Mint. You have yourself an awesome Blackberry Mojito.

INGREDIENTS

6 ounces blackberries

4 fresh mint leaves

1 lime, cut into 4 wedges

Mojito sparkling water or clear berry-flavored carbonated water

DIRECTIONS

Muddle one-quarter of the blackberries and mint leaves in each of the four glasses; squeeze a lime wedge over each glass and add ice. Top with the sparkling or carbonated water.

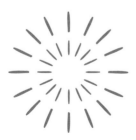

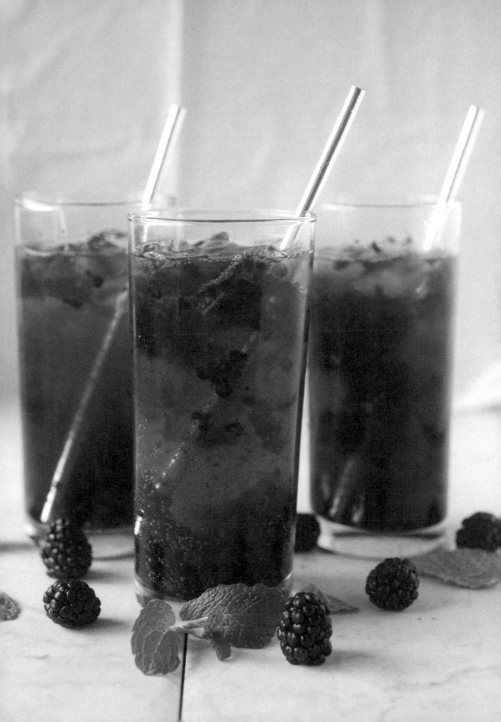

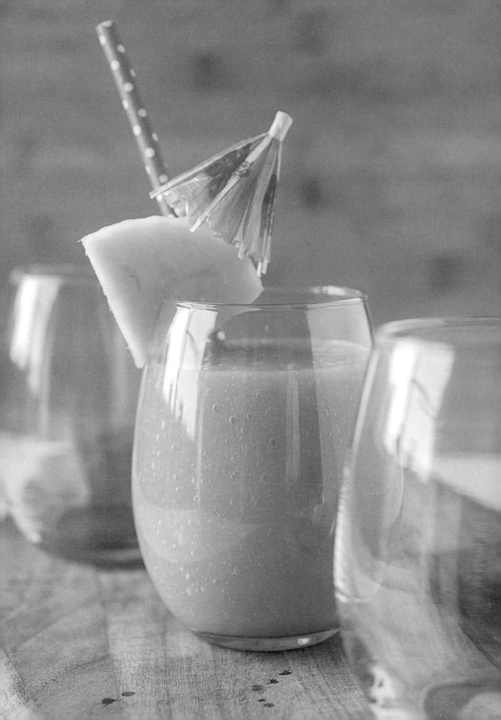

Mango and Papaya Fresca

YIELD: 4 servings

I have never had a fresca until this mocktail. Let me tell you
something: a fresca is the coolest and one of the most refreshing
beverages there is. You simply add your fruit to a blender
along with some cold water and blend! It's that easy! You can
get as creative with this fresca as you want; however, I highly
recommend you stick with the mango and papaya in this case.
It is just a delicious combination.

INGREDIENTS
½ ripe papaya, cut into chunks
3 large mangoes, cut into chunks
1¼ cups cold water
2 ounces Simple Syrup (page 22)

DIRECTIONS
Place the fruit, water, and simple syrup in a blender. Pulse until well
mixed. Pour into four glasses and serve.

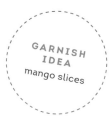

GARNISH
IDEA
mango slices

Orange Mimosa

YIELD: **2 servings**

An Orange Mimosa . . . it's the breakfast beverage. Nuff said.

INGREDIENTS

Juice of 4 large navel oranges
Orange-flavored carbonated water

DIRECTIONS

Pour the orange juice equally between the two champagne flutes and top off with the orange-flavored carbonated water.

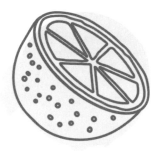

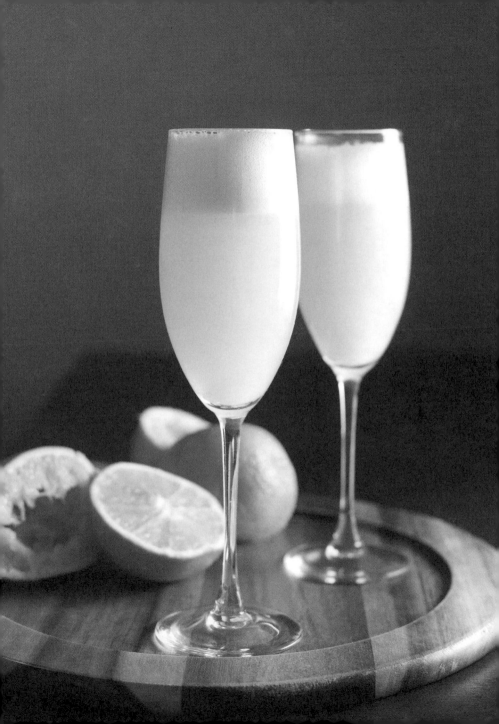

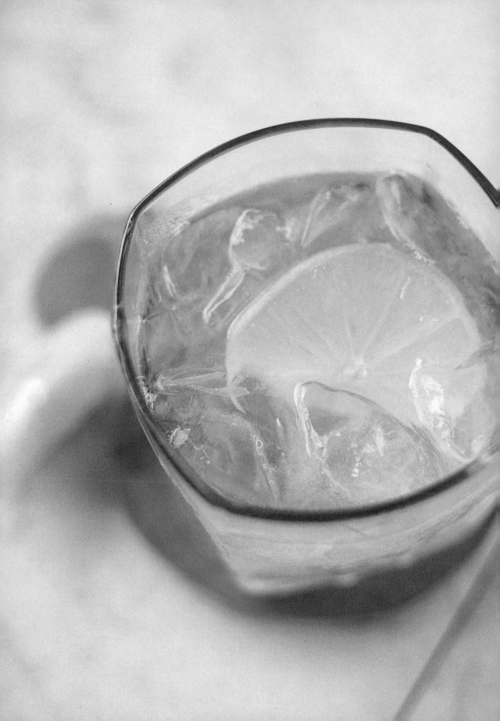

Virgin Tom Collins

YIELD: 1 serving

This is one of those cocktails that I see businessmen drink at the bars and I constantly think, "Why?" What is so important and great about gin, lime, and club soda? I am more of a sweet cocktail gal, so I don't think I will ever understand that concept. However, if they taste anything like this, I might be able to get with the program.

INGREDIENTS

Juice of ½ lime

Juice of ½ lemon

1 ounce Simple Syrup (page 22)

Club soda

GARNISH
IDEAS
lime or
lemon wedge

DIRECTIONS

Fill a small glass with ice, add the lime and lemon juice and the simple syrup, and top with club soda.

Frozen Peach Bellini

YIELD: **4 servings**

I want to drink this with my breakfast and brunch every time.
I love this drink so much, probably because peaches are my
favorite fruit. Oh, yes, when peaches are in season I am in the
grocery store every week, buying a bunch. So, to have them in a
glass . . . to drink . . . man, it is the best thing in the world to me.
What would make this Peach Bellini even better is to use fresh
peaches, if you can. Just slice them and put them in the freezer
until you are ready to use.

INGREDIENTS
5 cups frozen peach slices
1 cup peach puree
Peach-flavored carbonated water

DIRECTIONS
Place the still-frozen peaches and puree in a blender and pulse on
high speed for 2 to 3 minutes, until smooth. Pour into your desired
cocktail glasses and top with peach-flavored carbonated water.

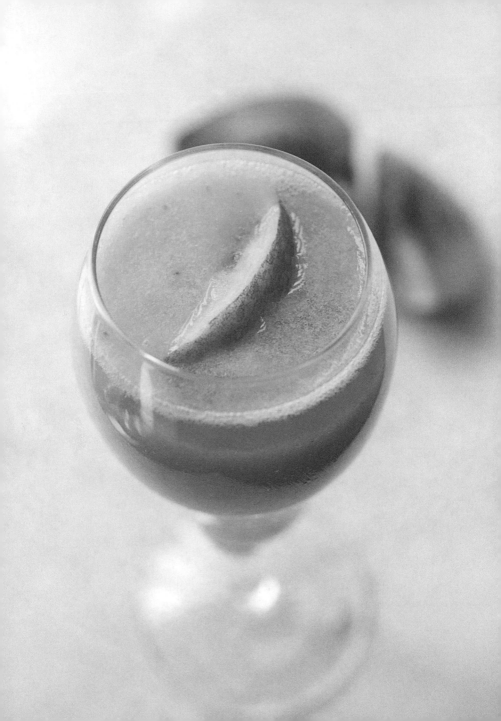

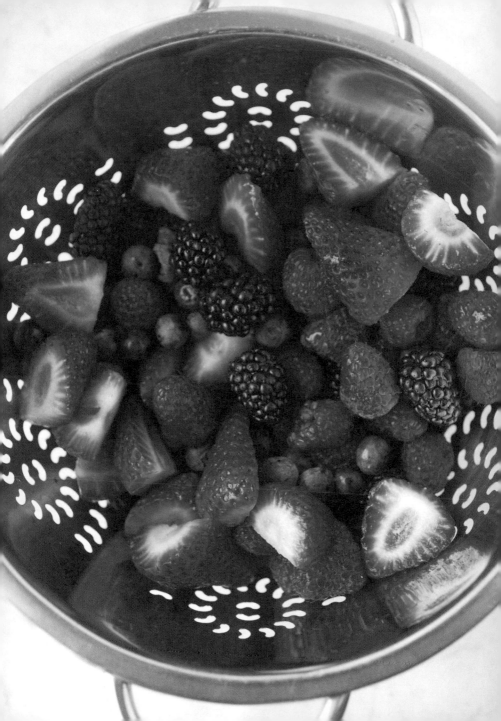

Berry Lemonade

YIELD: **1 gallon**

Okay . . . this is one of my favorite drinks in this entire book.
No kidding, I drank a gallon of this lemonade in two days. Yes,
it is that good. I was pleasantly surprised. I cannot wait until
the weather warms up, giving me a good excuse to make it again.
It is insanely delicious and refreshing. I know you will love it.

INGREDIENTS

1 pound strawberries, hulled

6 ounces blackberries

1 pint blueberries

6 ounces raspberries

Juice of 8 to 10 large lemons

1 cup Simple Syrup (page 22)

½ cup sugar

7 cups water

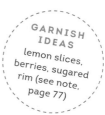

GARNISH
IDEAS
lemon slices,
berries, sugared
rim (see note,
page 77)

DIRECTIONS

Place the berries in a blender and pulse until smooth. Pour the
berry mixture into a gallon-size pitcher of your choice, add the
lemon juice, simple syrup, sugar, and water, and stir. Pour over ice
to serve.

Watermelon and Strawberry Cooler

YIELD: 4 servings

This is a recipe that is on my blog, and I love it so much I thought I'd share it with you. A few years ago I lost 30 pounds by eating right and exercising. I remember wanting something refreshing to drink without a lot of sugar, so I blended some watermelon, kiwi, and strawberries together and came up with this deliciousness! The added sweetener is a packet of stevia.

INGREDIENTS

8 cups watermelon chunks
1 pint strawberries, hulled and halved
2 kiwis, peeled and cut into fourths
One 1-ounce packet stevia
½ cup cold water

DIRECTIONS

Place the watermelon, strawberries, kiwi, stevia, and water in a blender and pulse until smooth. Serve in your desired glasses.

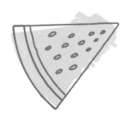

GARNISH IDEAS
fresh mint leaves, strawberries, and kiwi slices

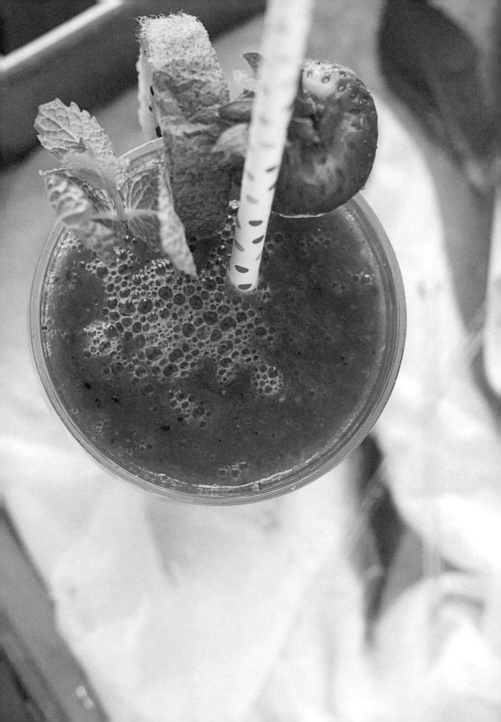

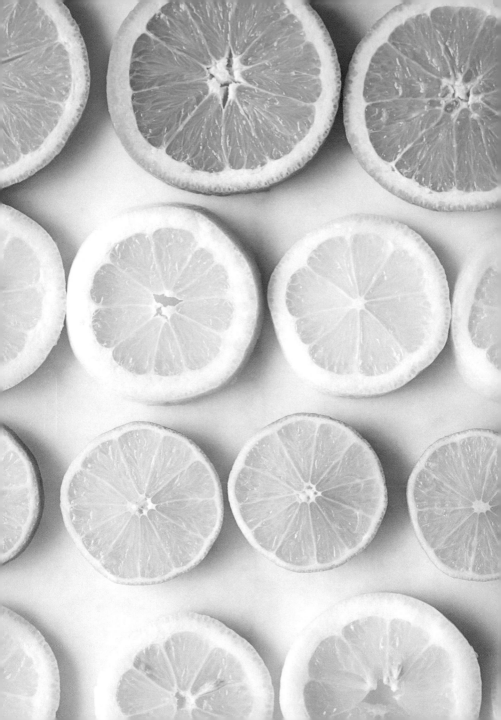

Citrus *and* White Tea Sangria

YIELD: **4 to 6 servings**

You are going to need something refreshing and crisp on the days when you're not feeling like yourself. A sangria filled with citrus fruit and a light and refreshing tea will do the trick.

INGREDIENTS

5 cups water

2 white tea bags

4 large navel oranges

4 large lemons

4 limes

2 fresh mint leaves

Lemon/lime-flavored carbonated water

3 ounces Simple Syrup (page 22)

GARNISH IDEAS
mint leaves; lemon, lime, and orange slices

Brew the tea in 5 cups of water. You will need strong tea for this recipe. Using a citrus juicer, juice 3 of the oranges, lemons, and limes. Slice the remaining orange, lemon, and lime. Fill a gallon pitcher halfway with ice and add the tea and citrus juice. Stir in the simple syrup and add the fruit slices and mint leaves to the pitcher. Refrigerate until ready to serve. Finish by adding the lemon/lime-carbonated water to fill the pitcher.

Red Hot Bomb

YIELD: **1 serving**

I loved Red Hots when I was younger. In fact, I still love the candy now. I am a sucker for cinnamon candies. I used to beg my grandmother to buy me a bag of the penny cinnamon candies at the drugstore when I was younger. Now I have found a way to enjoy my cinnamon craving without the cavities.

INGREDIENTS

5 ounces brewed chai tea
1.5 ounces Cinnamon Simple Syrup (page 23)
Pinch of ground cinnamon
Dash of grenadine

DIRECTIONS

Fill a small glass with ice and add the chai tea, cinnamon simple syrup, and cinnamon. Place a cup that is larger than the opening over the glass and shake well Add the grenadine and serve.

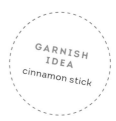

GARNISH IDEA
cinnamon stick

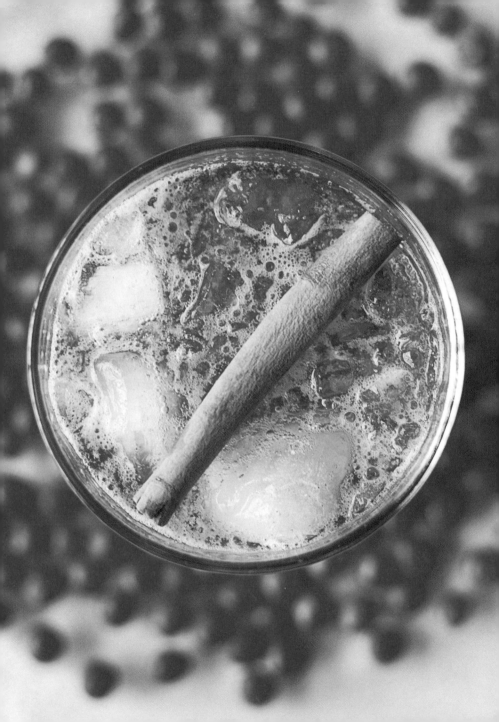

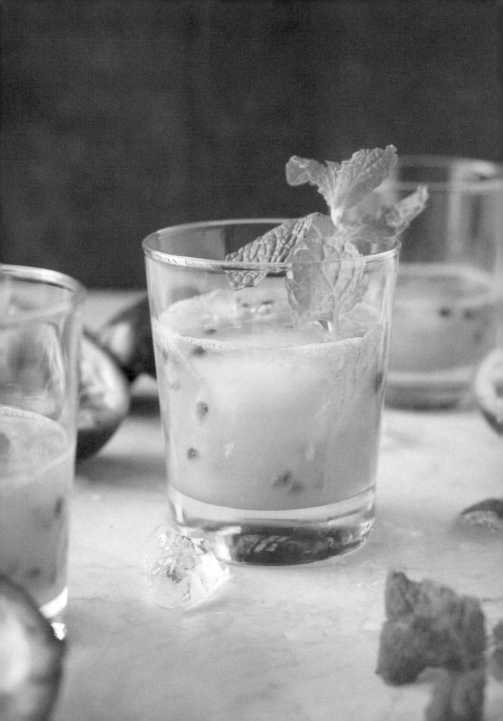

Passion Fruit Julep

YIELD: 4 servings

As I mentioned before, I absolutely love passion fruit! It is the best fruit (next to my peaches) on the face of the planet. I can eat a few pieces of passion fruit every day. With this drink, I'm sure I'll have you enjoying them daily, too!

INGREDIENTS
4 passion fruits
2.5 ounces Simple Syrup (page 22)
Club soda

DIRECTIONS
Scoop the insides of the passion fruit into a blender and add the simple syrup. Pulse for 1 to 2 minutes, until the fruit seems to have liquefied. Fill four small glasses with ice and divide the passion fruit mixture equally among the glasses. Top off with club soda.

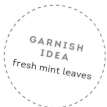

GARNISH
IDEA
fresh mint leaves

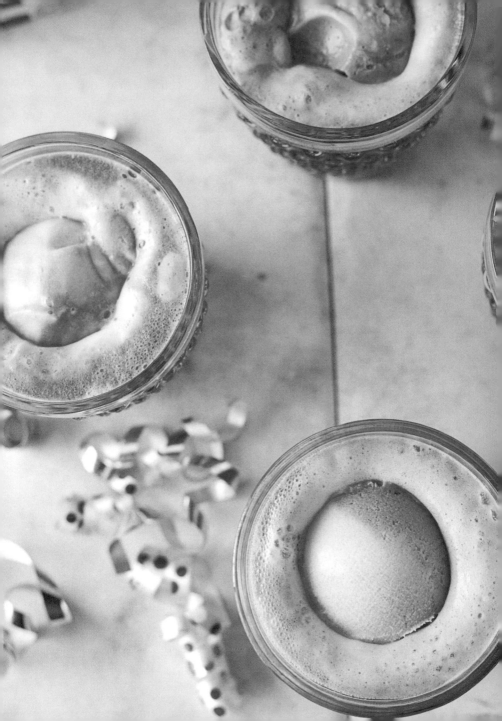

CHAPTER 3
SOMETHING SWEET

- -

The Third Trimester

OKAY, SO YOU MADE IT THIS FAR AND YOU'RE ALMOST READY TO MEET YOUR SWEET BUNDLE OF JOY. AREN'T YOU EXCITED?
You're probably noticing that although you feel good at times, you get tired very quickly, and sleep like a horse. It's as if you feel fine one minute and extremely exhausted the next. Your body hurts all the time; you can't get comfortable, no matter what you do; and your feet are tight and swollen. Oh, don't forget about those midnight leg cramps. I told you that your last three months are going to be difficult. Just keep in mind, this is the great sacrifice women must go through to bring forth our beautiful children! I must tell you that in case you don't feel that the payoff is worth it, but I promise it is. When you have finally given birth and you look down at that person that your body housed for nine months, you are going to immediately forget about the cravings, leg cramps, morning sickness, and fatigue. You're going to be too busy loving and kissing that baby that you have fallen in love with.

Third Trimester Checklist

 REST. A Lot of people are probably telling you that you need to get all the sleep you can now because when your baby gets here, you won't sleep as much. Although that is true, let me tell you, it won't matter how much sleep you get now; you are still going to be tired when that baby gets here. So, rest right now for you. Rest because what was once the size of a blueberry is growing into the size of a watermelon, and that is taking a toll on your body. Plus, you don't want to do too much, which could cause you to deliver early.

PACK YOUR BAGS. I recommend this for you and your significant other. Be sure to pack things that you will need, such as PJs, going-home outfits for you and your baby, toiletries, candles or whatever relaxes you, an iPod, house shoes or slippers, and whatever else you, your significant other, and baby will need to feel comfortable during your stay at the hospital.

TAKE BABY CLASSES. My husband and I took the basic baby-care class and the baby CPR class. We wanted to arm ourselves with as much knowledge as possible to prepare for our baby. I highly recommend that you take these classes, too, and if you are planning on breast-feeding, please take a breast-feeding class, as that information can be very helpful as well. Also, take a tour of the hospital so you can find out where you will be staying and where to direct your family and friends when your baby arrives.

 PUT EVERYTHING TOGETHER. I was so tired of putting together baby furniture that if I had to put together a box right now, I might cry. Work together with your partner to make sure everything is in working order and assembled properly. Also, be sure to put your baby's furniture exactly where you want it in the house, so you do not have to do any pulling or pushing when you get home. Everything will already be where you want it.

GET A MASSAGE. This is where I highly recommend spending some money and having a day at the spa. If you are anything like me, you don't feel particularly sexy or pretty. So do something that will help with that. Go to the spa, get pretty, get a manicure and pedicure, buy a cute maternity outfit, or do all the above. You've earned it. Wrap your mind around the fact that your body is making a human. I mean a person who is going to be walking, laughing, talking, thinking, and will grow up to be a contributing member of society someday. Your body is going through a lot, so be good to it.

 STRETCH. I would love to tell you that I worked out often during my pregnancy, but I didn't. However, I did do yoga a few times during my pregnancy and I felt so good afterward that I wanted to keep doing it. Your body is going through so much stress and tension, no matter how happy you may be feeling. Again, you're carrying a human being. Stretching will not only help you when it comes to delivery, but it also helps with healthy blood circulation.

NEST. I cleaned my house like no one's business. I got our carpets cleaned, washed the linens and all our laundry, wiped down my baby's room, cleaned the refrigerator, rearranged the cupboards, wiped down the baseboards and walls. That was just round one. You will go through something like this. But if your pregnancy is high risk, I would consider calling a cleaning service or having your family and friends do a task or two when they can.

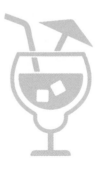

Brownie Affogato Sundae

YIELD: 1 serving

I love this sundae. It tastes amazing! You might think coffee over brownies wouldn't taste so great, but you'd be wrong. It makes the brownies and ice cream more decadent and delicious.

INGREDIENTS

1 brownie
1 scoop vanilla gelato
1 shot brewed espresso
Whipped cream
Chocolate shavings

DIRECTIONS

Crumble the brownie into the bottom of a coffee mug or your desired glass. Add the gelato, pour the espresso on top of the gelato, and top with whipped cream and chocolate shavings.

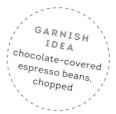

GARNISH IDEA
chocolate-covered espresso beans, chopped

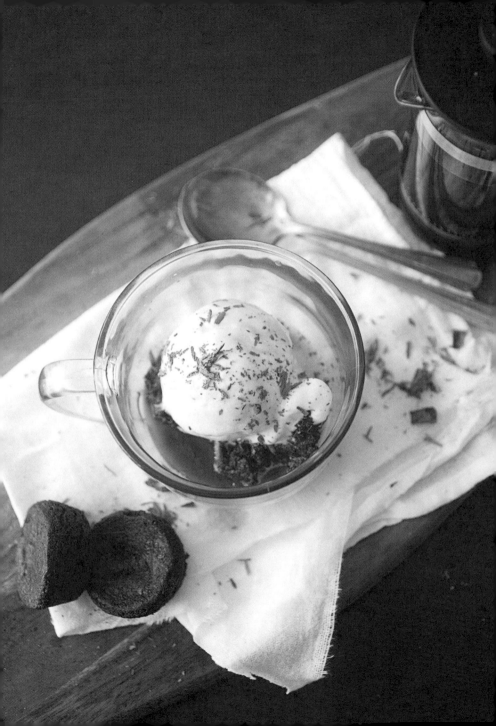

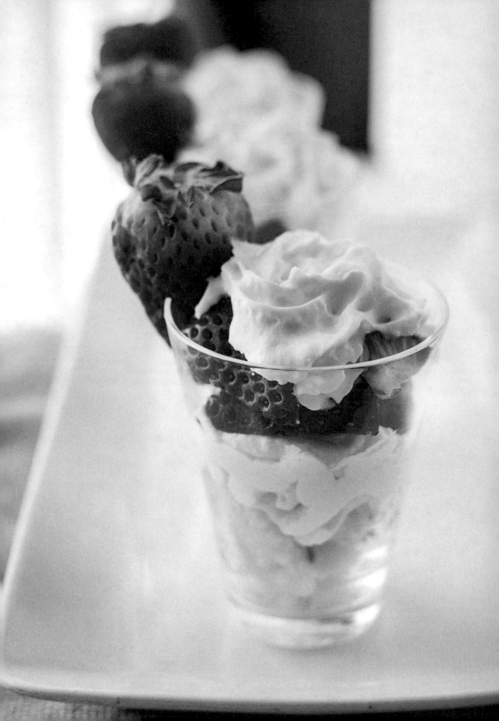

Strawberry Shortcake Shooters

YIELD: **4 servings**

These are perfectly small treats that you will love at any stage of your pregnancy. These deconstructed Strawberry Shortcake Shooters are so tempting and amazing.

INGREDIENTS

4 ounces cream cheese, at room temperature
2 tablespoons powdered sugar
1 teaspoon vanilla extract
1 cup hulled and diced strawberries
Four ½-inch slices pound cake
Whipped cream

DIRECTIONS

Crumble the slices of pound cake and add about 1 tablespoon of the crumbled cake into the bottom of four shot glasses. Set aside. Place the cream cheese, powdered sugar, and vanilla in a medium bowl and cream together until smooth. Spoon about 1 tablespoon of the cream cheese mixture in each shot glass, top with diced strawberries, and finish with whipped cream. Chill until ready to serve.

Raspberry Lemon Pops

YIELD: **4 pops**

The combination of sweet raspberries and tart lemon in these pops makes me all types of happy.

INGREDIENTS
12 ounces raspberries
Zest and juice of 1 large lemon
½ cup sugar

DIRECTIONS
Place the raspberries, lemon zest, and juice in a blender. Pulse until well blended. Pour the raspberry mixture through a fine-mesh strainer to remove the seeds. Pour into four ice pop molds and freeze for 6 to 8 hours or overnight.

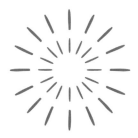

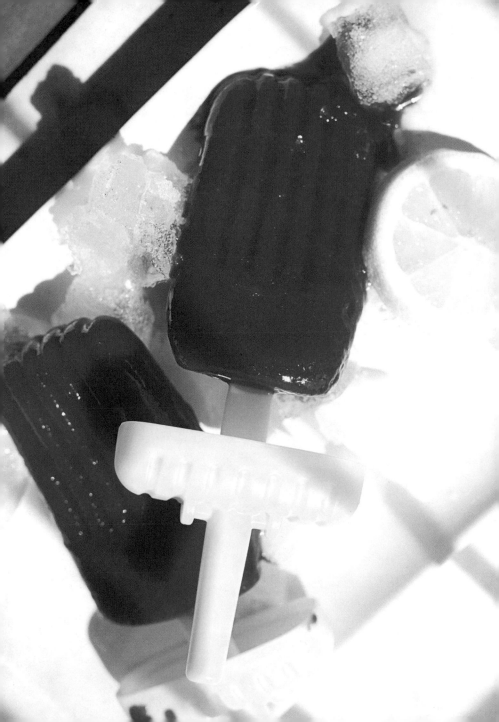

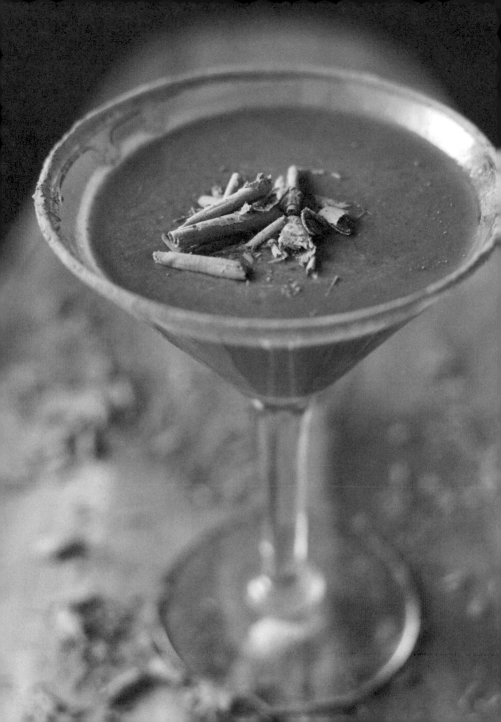

Spicy Chocolate Martini

YIELD: **2 servings**

Now, I need you to trust me on this one. You're going to see cayenne pepper in this martini, but do not let that scare you. In fact, the spiciness doesn't creep in until after you've enjoyed a sip. The spice isn't just in the cayenne—it's in the cinnamon as well. You'll love this martini.

INGREDIENTS

1 cup semisweet chocolate chips

½ cup heavy cream

2 ounces soy milk

3 ounces heavily brewed chai tea

1 ounce Cinnamon Simple Syrup (page 23)

Pinch of cayenne pepper

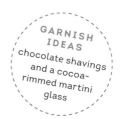

GARNISH IDEAS
chocolate shavings and a cocoa-rimmed martini glass

DIRECTIONS

Place the chocolate chips in a heat-safe bowl. Bring the heavy cream to a boil in a separate small saucepan and pour on top of the chocolate chips. Use a rubber spatula to stir until smooth; allow to cool.

Place the chocolate mixture, soy milk, brewed chai tea, the cinnamon simple syrup, and the cayenne and cinnamon in a shaker. Shake vigorously for 1 minute. Pour into two martini glasses and serve.

Honeydew and Cucumber Granita

I have always loved shaved lemon Italian ice. Have you ever had that before? It is super sweet, tart, and amazing. If you like shaved ice, you will love this recipe.

INGREDIENTS

1 honeydew melon

1 cucumber

1 lime

2 fresh mint leaves

½ cup Simple Syrup (page 22)

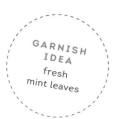

GARNISH IDEA
fresh mint leaves

DIRECTIONS

Cut the honeydew into chunks, removing the seeds and the skin. Remove the skin and seeds from the cucumber as well, and cut into slices.

Combine the honeydew melon, cucumber, mint leaves, and simple syrup in a food processor. Pulse until smooth. Place into a freezer container and freeze overnight. Use a fork to scrape the mixture. Place in your desired serving bowls.

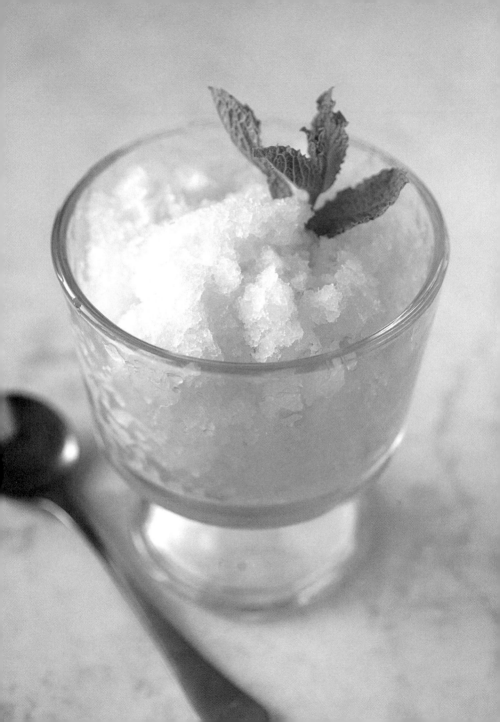

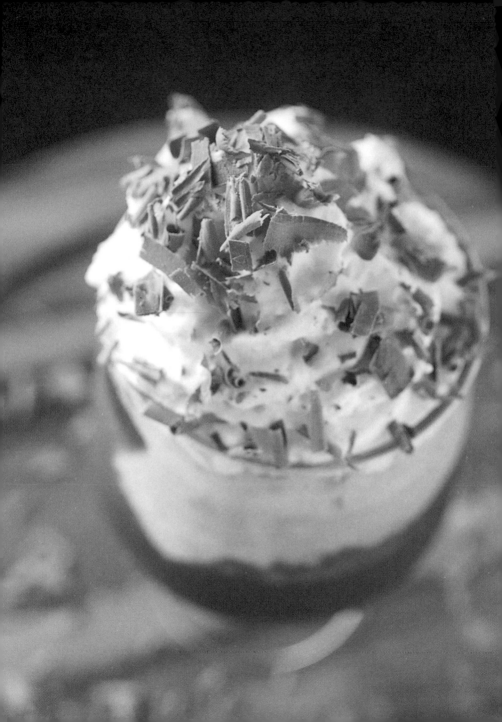

Black and White Mudslide

YIELD: **2 servings**

Mudslides are the perfect combination of coffee, ice cream, and chocolate. This milk shake may not have Kahlúa and Baileys Irish Cream, but it does have Baileys Syrup to give the taste and the illusion of these flavors. This is a super-smooth dessert drink.

INGREDIENTS
2 scoops vanilla ice cream
4 tablespoons Baileys Syrup
4 tablespoons brewed coffee
½ cup milk
2 scoops chocolate ice cream
¼ cup chocolate syrup

GARNISH IDEAS
whipped cream and chocolate shavings

DIRECTIONS

Combine the vanilla ice cream, 2 tablespoons of the Baileys Syrup, 2 tablespoons of the coffee, and ¼ cup of the milk in a blender. Pour in a large glass and set aside. Repeat, using the chocolate ice cream and the remaining syrup, coffee, and milk, and pour in a second large glass. Pour half of the chocolate syrup into an individual serving glass in a circular motion to coat, and then alternate pouring in the chocolate and vanilla ice cream until ¾ full and finish with fresh whipped cream.

NOTE: Add more ice cream while blending, if desired, to reach the thickness you desire.

Apple Pie Milk Shake

YIELD: 1 serving

I know this is such a crazy concept to you, but let me confirm that
I did add a whole slice of apple pie to a blender and turned it into a
milk shake. You can do this to just about any pie, but let's start with
apple pie first.

INGREDIENTS

1 slice apple pie
½ cup milk
2 to 3 scoops vanilla ice cream
2 tablespoons caramel sauce
Pinch of ground cinnamon

PIECRUST STRIPS

1 prebaked piecrust
2 tablespoons unsalted butter
Cinnamon sugar

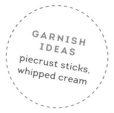

GARNISH IDEAS
piecrust sticks,
whipped cream

DIRECTIONS

Place slice of pie, milk, ice cream, caramel, and cinnamon in a
blender. Blend until smooth. Pour into your desired glass.

To make the piecrust strips: cut the piecrust into medium strips,
brush slightly with the butter, and sprinkle with the cinnamon
sugar. Bake at 350°F for 10 minutes, or until crisp. Use to garnish
the milk shake.

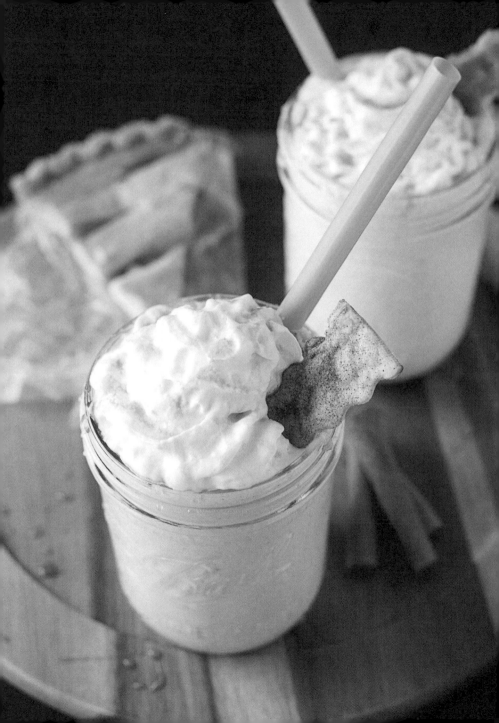

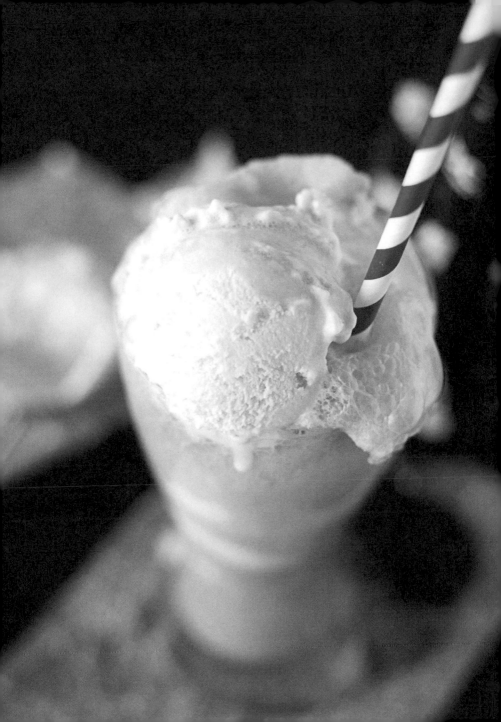

Classic Root Beer Float

No one loves root beer like me and no one loves root beer floats as much as I do. Root beer was love at first taste for me. During the final stages of my pregnancy, this was an amazing treat that was well deserved.

INGREDIENTS

2 scoops vanilla ice cream

One 12-ounce can or bottle root beer

DIRECTIONS

Place the ice cream in a tall glass, fill halfway with the root beer, and serve.

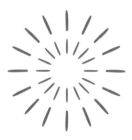

Baby Shower Punch

YIELD: **Varies**

I have this punch at every event, family holiday, and baby shower! I don't know whether this is an official recipe, but I decided to make it official. This is a super-fun punch that you must have at your baby shower and should have at every party. All you need is a punch bowl; pour in the ingredients and you have yourself a party in a bowl.

INGREDIENTS

Fruit punch
Pineapple juice
Lemon-lime soda
Rainbow sherbet

DIRECTIONS

Pour equal parts fruit punch, pineapple juice, and lemon-lime soda into a large punch bowl. Float scoops of rainbow sherbet on top of the punch. Set out to serve.

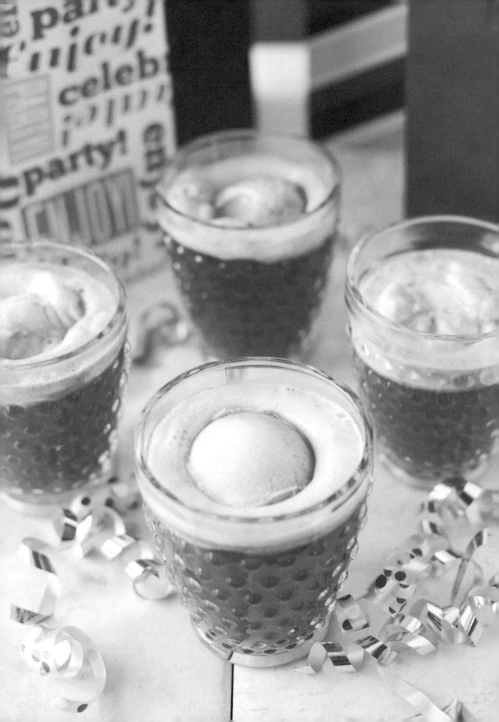

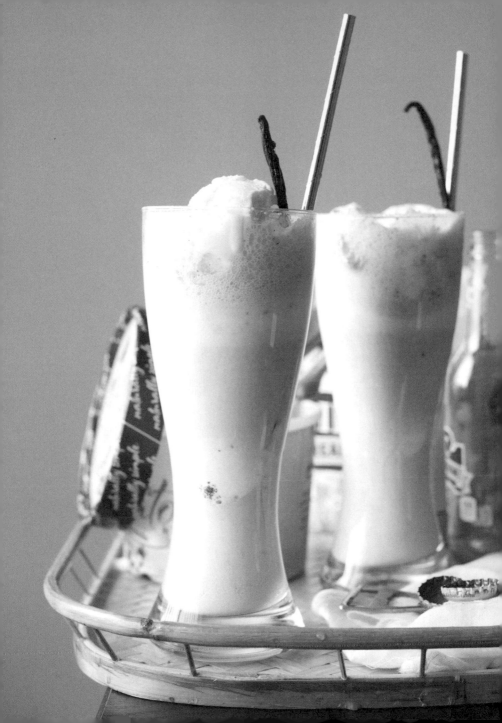

Vanilla Bean Cream Soda Float

YIELD: **2 servings**

You can tell that I am a sucker for floats. I love cream soda just as much as I love root beer. To make these cream soda floats even more delicious, I've added the scrapings of the vanilla bean to enhance that smooth vanilla flavor. Can't find vanilla beans? No worries, just continue with the cream soda and vanilla ice cream. This float will still rock your boat.

INGREDIENTS
2 vanilla beans
One 12-ounce bottle cream soda
2 scoops vanilla ice cream

DIRECTIONS
Slice the vanilla beans in half lengthwise, using a sharp knife. Use the back of the knife to scrape out the insides. Place the insides of the vanilla beans into two of your preferred serving glasses; add a little cream soda, and use a whisk to break up the vanilla. Add a scoop of ice cream to each glass and pour the rest of the cream soda to the top of the glasses. Add more ice cream if desired. Serve with a straw or spoon.

Blackberry and Chocolate Panna Cotta

YIELD: **4 servings**

Panna cotta is a smooth and decadent dessert that is a perfect after-dinner treat. You ease on down the glass through the layers of blackberry custard to the best part—the chocolate custard! This is super easy and delicious. You will love it.

INGREDIENTS

3 cups heavy cream
Two ¼-ounce envelopes unflavored gelatin, divided
½ cup mascarpone cheese
5 tablespoons sugar
2 teaspoons salt
3 ounces semisweet chocolate, chopped
18 ounces blackberries
1 tablespoon orange zest
1 tablespoon orange juice

GARNISH IDEAS
blackberries and chocolate shavings

DIRECTIONS

Combine ¼ cup of the cream and one envelope of gelatin in a small, heatproof bowl. Set aside and allow to thicken. Once firm, place over boiling water and stir to allow the gelatin to dissolve.

Meanwhile, place 1¼ cups of the cream along with ¼ cup of the mascarpone, 2 tablespoons of the sugar, and 1 teaspoon of the salt in a medium saucepan and bring to a boil. Once dissolved, remove from the heat. Add the chocolate and stir until dissolved

continued

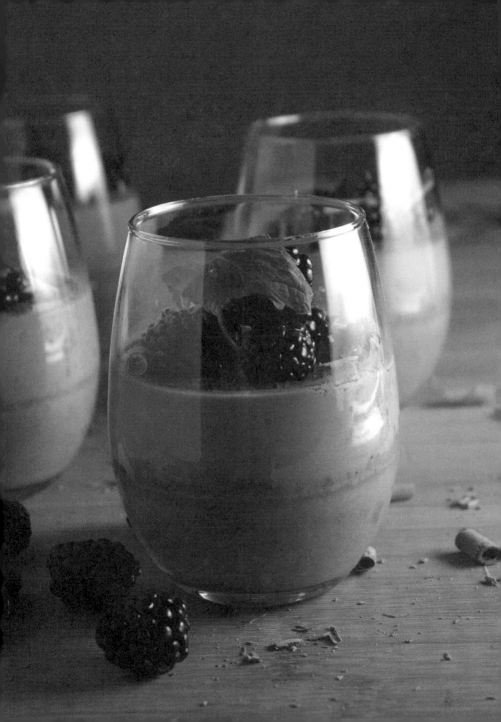

and smooth. Next, add the gelatin mixture to the chocolate mixture and stir. Using a fine-mesh strainer, strain the chocolate mixture into a pourable measuring cup. Divide the chocolate mixture equally among four serving glasses. Place in the refrigerator for at least 3 hours, or until the chocolate becomes firm.

When ready to assemble the panna cotta, rinse and dry the small, heatproof bowl. Combine ¼ cup of the cream and with the remaining envelope of gelatin in the bowl. Heat the same way as before, over boiling water, to dissolve.

Meanwhile, place the blackberries, orange zest, orange juice, and 1 tablespoon of the remaining sugar in a medium saucepan. Bring to a simmer and allow the blackberries to break down, about 10 minutes. Use a masher to smash the berries. Use a fine-mesh strainer to remove any seeds and strain the blackberries into a pourable measuring cup.

Place the remaining 1¼ cups of cream, ¼ cup of mascarpone, 2 tablespoons of sugar, and teaspoon of salt in a medium saucepan and bring to a boil. Once dissolved, remove from the heat. Pour in the blackberry mixture and the gelatin mixture and stir. Pour evenly on top of the firmed chocolate panna cotta. Place back in the refrigerator and allow to chill and become firm for at least 3 hours or overnight.

ACKNOWLEDGMENTS

I guess the first entity I should acknowledge is Mother Nature herself. If it wasn't for her cruel joke of making me CRAVE alcohol while I was pregnant, I would not have had the motivation or creative space to make the drinks in this book. So, thank you Mother Nature, for loving and hating me at the same time; this book may not have been possible with your bipolar personality.

Then there is the child that was growing inside me during this tortuous time of my life. You are an amazing gift from God that I will never take for granted. I promise to continue to pursue you, encourage you, and try to not screw you up too badly in the process. Once you are old enough to read this book, please know that you are goofy because you have inherited that part of your personality from both of your parents, and not from the alcohol I so often wanted to consume. I promise!

My loving and mothering mother. Can you believe this?! Did you know, when you were carrying me in your womb, that you would give birth to a child with the task of changing the world in a very specific way? To become a published cookbook author and blogger? Who knew?! You have groomed me and molded me to

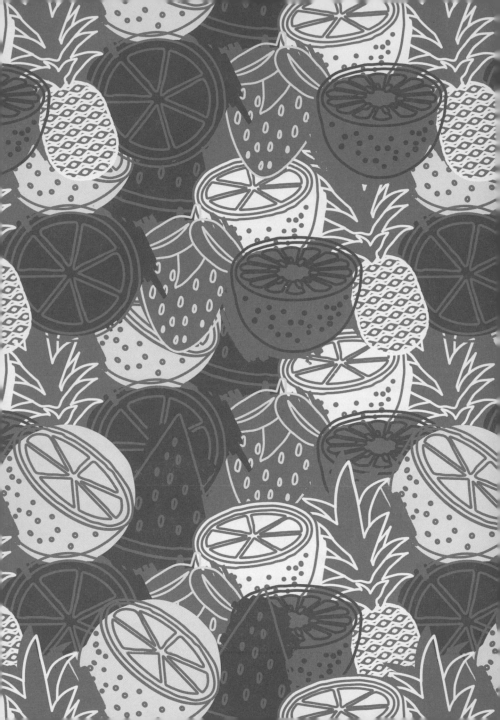

go after things in life that no one else could possibly understand except you. It's crazy how you get my crazy. Please keep encouraging me to think and dream crazy!

To my friends, who have been along for the Brown Sugar ride from the very beginning: Kim, "Murray," Dayana, Sarah, Cynthia, Angela, Rachel (for making a bomb logo), my brothers (Frank, John, and Michael), Mojo, countless cousins, and other friends and family members.

To everyone at The Countryman Press, especially Ann Treistman, for believing in this book and making it happen! Ann, thank you for finding me. You have made one of my dreams come true and I sincerely hope you and I can continue working together.

For anyone that I am forgetting, as my loving Paw-Paw Bizzell would say, charge it to my head, not my heart.

To my heartbeat, my lawyer, my confidant, my best friend, my pastor, my homie, my prayer partner, my lover, my foundation, my husband. I know, without a doubt, that if it weren't for you, I would not have been given the opportunity to make this book and my blog would be crap. I must've given up on myself one hundred times, questioning why I even blog in the first place, and why can't I be happy with a job. You somehow manage to see something in me that I can't. Since 2012, you have told me that something amazing is going to come from my blog and, even when I thought you were crazy, I dared to believe you. You have never let me give up or give in and I will always be eternally grateful to you for pushing me. Words have not yet been created that will give depth to my deepest gratitude and adoration for you being in my life. I love you, dude!

Lastly, to all my family members who cannot be here to physically witness this milestone, Daisy Nared, Frank Nared Sr., Frank Nared Jr., Mattie Bizzell, Calvin "Roc" Washington, "Cookie," and Susie Minter. Most importantly, my firstborn son, Shaun DeMarcus Weaver. I breathe your memory every day; I carry your warmth in my heart; and I carry your smile in my spirit. I miss you and love you every day and I hope that I made you proud.

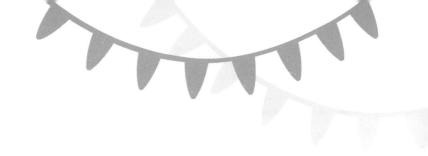

INDEX

ABOUT
THE AUTHOR

Hello, Sugar Babies! What is a "Sugar Baby"? You are now, but to be more specific, "Sugar Babies" is what I call my blog followers. My name is Nicole, and I have been a food blogger for five years! My blog, *Brown Sugar: A City Girl Making Life Look Sexy*, came out of absolute boredom. That may be hard to believe, but it is true. In my late 20s I was super bored with life and had nothing else to do but watch Netflix and bake a bunch of things I had never baked before. It all started with the Matcha Green Tea Cupcakes I made for a company potluck. I had never made them before and I wanted to impress my colleagues by baking something more than Funfetti Cupcakes from a box. Without any expectation of how my newfound love of baking would be received, my Matcha Green Tea Cupcakes were a huge hit, so I decided to continue baking. I started baking so much, I decided to take pictures of what I was making and post the recipes on a blog as a way of keeping track of everything. Along with that, I kept a journal of my thoughts and stories that I associated with whatever I made, and I soon realized that, without my knowing, I was blogging. From there came writing about my experiences with dating, getting engaged, getting married, and now being a mom. The lesson in this

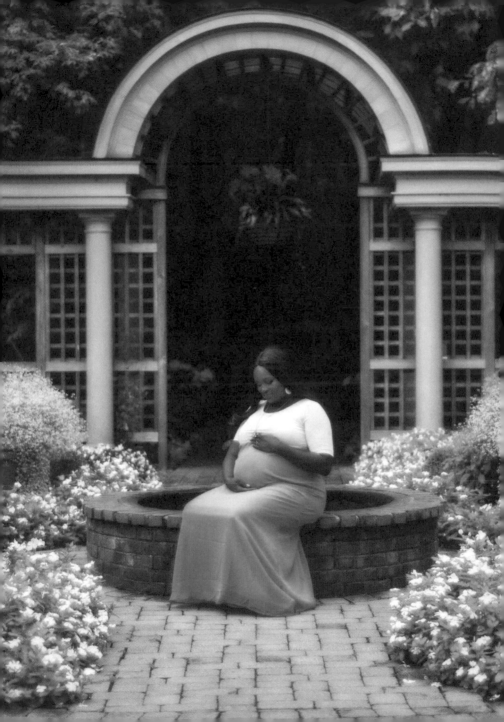

overview of how I started blogging is not to inspire you to start baking, but to encourage you to never pass on an interest that comes out of boredom, as you never know where it will take you.

In the beginning, I spent a lot of time thinking about the type of blogger and blog I wanted. I didn't want another dessert blog and I didn't want a blog that was only full of recipes. I wanted to write about topics that would (hopefully) get people engaged and ignite conversation about topics I was passionate about. At the time, I was passionate about sharing my experiences with dating. I would pose rhetorical questions about love and relationships in hopes of beginning a dialogue about some of the challenges we all have experienced while dating and being in a relationship. I considered myself to be an extension of Carrie Bradshaw, from my favorite show, *Sex and the City*. I wanted to create a space where people could get delicious recipes and find something entertaining and thought provoking to read. While writing about my love life, I also began podcasting about various subjects surrounding love and dating. I have created a space in the blogosphere where people feel they are going to a friend's house for an amazing dinner and stimulating conversation. I hope you visit my blog and join me at my table, where I make delicious food and discuss mommy woes, the joys and trials of marriage and dating, and relationships.

For information about special discounts for bulk
purchases, please contact W. W. Norton Special Sales
at specialsales@wwnorton.com or 800-233-4830

Manufacturing by Versa Press
Book design by LeAnna Weller Smith
Production manager: Devon Zahn

The Countryman Press
www.countrymanpress.com

A division of W. W. Norton & Company, Inc.
500 Fifth Avenue, New York, NY 10110
www.wwnorton.com

978-1-68268-154-1 (pbk.)

10 9 8 7 6 5 4 3 2 1

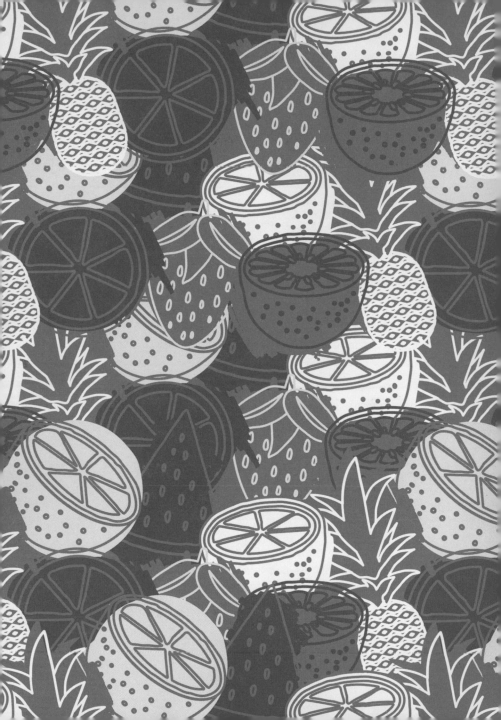